ENDORSEMENTS

"The first thing that is apparent about Frank Shelton is his passion for Christ. The second thing is that he really cares about people and wants us to understand the life-changing mysteries of the Kingdom of God. When a seemingly insignificant life is surrendered wholly to our great God, then the so-called impossible becomes a way of life. Welcome to the great adventure!"

Sheila Walsh, author of "The Storm Inside"
"Women of Faith" conference speaker/singer
and former co-host "700 Club"

"My friend Frank is a man on fire. He has one thing to say: Jesus Christ loves you no matter what. This book is an incredible reminder to those who have a relationship with Christ and an incredible informer to those seeking Christ that He made you already with Greatness. Greatness comes to light when we believe and obey what God tells us to do. I couldn't think of a better person then Frank Shelton, Jr. to write about how we as humans were born with Greatness instilled in us. He is truly the most encouraging person that I have ever met. Frank is a gifted author, a phenomenal teacher and a voice of truth and encouragement that
truly blesses my soul."

Graham Antony Tchividjian - Young Entrepreneur and grandson of Rev. Billy Graham

"Frank Shelton has a rare and powerful gift of using words to inspire people to unearth their potential. If you have ever had the pleasure of hearing Frank speak as I have on several occasions (Dallas, TX, London, England and Brazil in 2016), you would know why you have to read his book, "Carrying Greatness." Frank has the gift of encouragement and he has been such a blessing to me. I am always eager to hear what Frank has to say because his words bring hope and healing."

Joe DeLoach - USA Gold Medalist - 200 M

"Frank Shelton, Jr has been motivational and inspirational in lives around the world for many years, including mine! He's been living my motto: "Changing Lives to Change the World." He connects with any audience and I would highly recommend Frank for any classroom, corporate or Christian Event. Frank and I have spoken together nearly a dozen times in five states and I have seen him in a variety of settings and he exudes Christ and class wherever he goes. He is the consummate people person and I asked him to write a foreword in my book "TRUST YOUR NEXT SHOT" along with Bill Cosby and Michael Jordan. I invited him as my personal guest to World Series Winner Albert Pujols banquet in St Louis and I could have selected anyone in the world and I picked him. Frank is a powerful presence, dynamic communicator and also a great comedian. It is my belief that "laughter is a great medicine!" He totally lives 'carrying greatness" and I'm honored to serve on the Winning Team with him. He is my friend and a leader to all."

Meadowlark Lemon - Basketball Hall of Fame,
Harlem Globetrotter & Child of God

"Frank Shelton's book, Carrying Greatness is a message of hope for this generation. Frank is the type of communicator who brings audiences laughter but also reminds every individual of the sacredness of the death and resurrection of our savior Jesus Christ. We live in a culture that is desperate for hope and Frank communicates a message of hope in Christ. Jesus specifically designed and created you. Some parents may believe "they made a mistake" regarding the birth of a child. But Frank reminds us that God makes NO mistakes. Even in sad cases of pregnancy that results from a one-night stand or rape, God still orchestrates good. The Bible says, "We know that God works all things together for good for those who love Him." Jesus ultimately designed you and made no mistakes with your body or mind. The Scripture says you are "God's work of art." Another translation says, "You are God's masterpiece." Each of us is a unique creation, a one-of-a-kind; and with God there is no shoddy workmanship, no junk. Because he lovingly created us and has ongoing plans for our lives, we can trust Him. King David wrote:

"For it was You (God) who created my inward parts;
You knit me together in my mother's womb.

I will praise you because I have been remarkably
and wonderfully made.
Your works are wonderful, and I know this very well."

Evangelist Frank Shelton reminds us that Jesus, the creator of the universe, designed us! This book, Carrying Greatness will inspire you to live for God; the One who's very Essence is Greatness! He made you and you are special—remarkably and wonderfully made because Jesus uniquely designed you. Because of this, you can trust Him. This doesn't mean that life isn't hard and full of temptations and sins. But we have hope in Jesus. In moments of disappointment, we can still focus on the goodness of God. King David, who suffered much rejection as a young man, kept his focus on the goodness of God. He wrote, "I would have despaired unless I had believed that I would see the goodness of the Lord in the land of the living." Paul told the church in Rome that God has the power to use even the bad things in our life to bring about good in some way. "And we know that in all things," he wrote, "God works for the good of those who love him, who have been called according to his purpose. God doesn't want us to settle for secondary pleasures that take us away from the greatest pleasure discovered in Him. Jesus said, "I come to that you they may have life and have it more abundantly."

    Dave Sterrett - Author/Co-author "I Am Second"
    & "Is the Bible True…Really?"

"Carrying Greatness" is not just motivational and inspirational it will arrest your heart! When I read Carrying Greatness, Sharing Greatness, Sparing Greatness and Wearing Greatness, I began to cry because the whole point of the book came into focus. The greatness God has placed inside every one of us is meant to impact the world and bring Him glory. It was then that I was struck with the responsibility and weight of the greatness we all carry. My prayer became God use all that is good in me to point others Lord to thee. Please forgive the rhyming prayer and let God speak to your heart as you read this book.

    Frank Santora - Lead Pastor, Faith Church CT & NYC
    Author – "After You Die" and "Turn It Around"
    TBN "Praise the Lord" host

CARRYING GREATNESS

FRANKLIN SHELTON, JR.

CONTENTS

DEDICATION

To my parents, Frank and Sharon Shelton who gave me life. My bride, Ruth who reminds me daily of God's grace and unconditional love. My children, Hannah Grace and Andrew Lincoln whom are on loan from Heaven and I love whole heartedly on Earth. My siblings, Matt and Jaime who make me smile on every remembrance of our youth and I'm proud of both of you as adults.

Shout out to all the anonymous heroes (past and present) who didn't have much fanfare but are winners the same and know your reward in Heaven is huge! Members of our armed forces who carry greatness daily as you represent our nation in your duties ensuring our freedom. MSgt Aaron Torian, USMC whom was recently laid to rest at Arlington National Cemetery for paying the ultimate price and we are indeed grateful for your service.

For every politician who stood up for the little guy and promoted Truth even at the expense of political re-election. Thank you to all clergy who unselfishly fed His sheep and each itinerant preacher who left loved ones throughout the centuries to travel the globe pointing complete strangers to a personal relationship with Christ to help enlarge the Family of God before it's eternally too late. Without a doubt you carry greatness each time you proclaim God's Holy Word.

Last but not least, thanks to my Creator and Savior who not only created us all in His image but deposited the Holy Spirit in the born again believer and with us each step of the way. May we walk worthy of Him because as kids of The King we never walk alone and each of us carry greatness.

WORD TO THE WISE

The Bible says repeatedly, "He that hath ears must listen." When the Master speaks we do well to listen. One can be smart and still not wise.

Jesus shared a parable in Matthew 25:14-30 "For it is just like a man about to go on a journey, who called his own slaves and entrusted his possessions to them. To one he gave five talents, to another, two, and to another, one, each according to his own ability; and he went on his journey. Immediately the one who had received the five talents went and traded with them, and gained five more talents. In the same manner the one who had received the two talents gained two more. But he who received the one talent went away, and dug a hole in the ground and hid his master's money. Now after a long time the master of those slaves came and settled accounts with them. The one who had received the five talents came up and brought five more talents, saying, 'Master, you entrusted five talents to me. See, I have gained five more talents.

His master said to him, 'Well done, good and faithful slave. You were faithful with a few things, I will put you in charge of many things; enter into the joy of your master. Also the one who had received the two talents came up and said, 'Master, you entrusted two talents to me. See, I have gained two more talents. His master said to him, 'Well done, good and faithful slave. You were faithful with a few things, I will put you in charge of many things; enter into the joy of your master. And the one also who had received the one talent came up and said, 'Master, I knew you to be a hard man, reaping where you did not sow and gathering where you scattered no seed. And I was afraid, and went away and hid your talent in the ground. See, you have what is yours. "But his master answered and said to him, 'You wicked, lazy slave, you knew that I reap where I did not sow and gather where I scattered no seed. Then you ought to have put my money in the bank, and on my arrival I would have received my money back with interest. Therefore take away the talent from him, and give it to the one who has the ten talents. "For to everyone who has, more shall be given, and he will have abundance; but from the one who does not have, even what he does have shall be taken away. Throw out the worthless slave into the outer darkness; in that place there will be weeping and gnashing of teeth."

We cannot work our way into Heaven but those born-again will be rewarded for their works. To think the Almighty will award crowns on behalf of Christ in the next life is exciting. All of us have been entrusted with gifts and talents that are deposited deep in us by Divinity and we have two options, *invest* them or *waste* them. One day we will stand and give an account to God for what we did or didn't do with those gifts. The Bible is clear "to whom much is given much is required (Luke 12:48)."

Someone shared with me years ago, "If God gave a friend five talents and another two and one to another. Truthfully, if the one came back returning only four of the five and the others returned with two and one, respectfully technically the two latter did more than the first."

Greatness is not cheap and some will admire and applaud you and others will try to destroy your gift and will long for your demise. It will inspire some and intimidate others but the key is to be thankful for both the Giver and gift. The Bible says, "Every good and perfect gift comes from above (James 1:17)." The Lord in Heaven embedded and invested in us on Earth with talents to glorify Him and assist others. Too often we are trying to compete with others when we should use our skills to compliment. We would do better not to "outdo" but out serve each other. Pastor Ed Young, Jr. said in a sermon, "If you are not serving than you are swerving."

While in London, England in 2012 during the Olympics I had the privilege to reunite and serve with my friend and Olympian Joe DeLoach. He won the gold medal for Team USA in 1988 at Seoul, Korea in 200M relay beating "Olympian of the Century" Carl Lewis. Carl had already won nine but his teammate took his tenth gold medal. Over a meal together, Joe shared with me that we have to run our own race. In track and field if we are to step in another's lane we are disqualified. Joe couldn't be Mother Teresa in some aspects of life and she in her prime couldn't beat him in a sprint. We need to run our race, stay in our lane, block out the crowd, keep our eyes on the prize and run to the very end for an Audience of One.

Those who think the grass is greener on the other side forget that a septic tank is somewhere close by. We need to be content in our calling and use our gifts and talents to benefit others not a burden to them. When we view others as colleagues not competition we all win. Unfortunately, we live in a fallen world and not everyone plays fair or with class. If there is one thing I have learned in my life it is that sometimes the greatest gifts come in super small packages. On countless game shows, I have seen eager contestants bypass the small for a much larger door or box only to get a gag gift or worse, a life-long supply of Chia Pets! Chia Pets are nice if you are a kid, but if, as an adult, you missed a brand new fully-equipped Kia automobile, it is a tad disappointing. Too often we go for the big and miss the "bigger" prize.

Over the years, I have also learned that the obvious isn't obvious. The guaranteed isn't always the 'sure thing'. Regardless, if out of jealousy or incompetency, the 'real deal' often is left on the shelf while cubic zirconias are promoted and purchased.

The great Charlie Chaplin heard of a contest with Charlie Chaplin impersonators coming from all over the country to compete for a prize. He thought it was comical and actually entered the contest himself. You could feel the electricity in the air! The place was packed with contestants sporting Chaplin's trademark mustache. Moments before it started, the contestants filed on stage and something peculiar happened.

Drum roll please......unbeknownst to the crowd, contestants or judges, would you believe that the real Charlie Chaplin came in THIRD place? How is that possible? Just another example of that in life, the obvious isn't always obvious! Keep in mind, that bigger is not always better and what may look like disappointments initially may be Divine Appointments eternally. Today, dare to look for the good in everyone! Give others the benefit of the doubt; celebrate the value of those with whom you come in contact. Try to be 'big' enough to compliment others and not be intimidated because of them. Perhaps most importantly, remember when you are bypassed or overlooked, don't take it personally. The very best eventually had their moments in the limelight, but they also knew the private pain of rejection and scorn along the way.

View future criticism as a compliment not a complaint. President Ronald Reagan said, "When you are kicked from behind it just means you are out front." Since most are too slow or small to compliment, they criticize instead. Throw a spin on it and keep walking forward, knowing you are on the right track. Remember, anyone can criticize but it takes class and competence to create.

May this book inspire you to never view life the same again. Our time on Earth is way too short to miss the value all around or the worth deposited deep inside of you. You are an original and don't dare try to be a carbon copy of someone else. No one can be you better than YOU! God makes no mistakes and you are priceless. Enjoy the journey!

May these individuals in the following chapters inspire you to not waste another day wondering if you are valuable? You are destined for greatness and the best is yet to come. Regardless, if you believe it or not, you are indeed carrying greatness. Get a grip on God's great grace and get moving, because the world is waiting to see the real you! My prayer is that you will not only realize that you have potential but you will also find your purpose and fall in love with the Person who created you.

Life is so much more than living and dying but rather dying to live for the One who gave His all for us and knowing Him intimately. My neighbors, who lived two doors down when I was a child, had a sign in their kitchen that stated: "Your life is God's gift to you, but what you do with your life is your gift to God." Indeed, you are great because God created you in His image and deposited greatness in you. On top of that the Son of God died on the cross as a payment for our sin. When you take His love and couple that with His grace you cannot lose. Greatness is in each and everyone one of us and let us not be the coward or crowd to bury it but the remnant who carry it and invests in others for His glory. Carry greatness and Greatness will carry you!

"A man's gift makes room for him, and brings him before great men and kings." (Proverbs 18:16)

CHAPTER ONE

SEEMS SO SMALL

William Easton worked for the U.S. Park Service and was a foreman. He had served faithfully for years and now with retirement looming, was entrusted with another assignment. In 1912, he was given the task to plant small seedlings in the ground all around Washington, D.C.

The catch is it was the coldest winter on record in the Nation's Capital and secondly, some of his colleagues were quite possibly complaining of this latest task convinced it just another menial job stuck outside in the cold. After all, the seedlings *seemed so small*. Not sure what is worse, the cold climate or chilling complaints from colleagues. Easton and his crew were instructed to plant them around the Tidal Basin and they learned they were a gift from another nation. Over the years, I have come to the conclusion that sometimes the biggest blessings come in the smallest bundles. What looked like an obstacle may be an unusual opportunity.

For several months, they embraced the cold and took their task to heart. They layered up with their warmest clothes and marched outside and got on their hands and knees and went to work. Working by day and into the night they were busy bees and nothing deterred their focus for a faithful and hopefully a fruitful finish. Equipped with a work ethic that didn't know quit and despite something so small in their hands initially they continued to plant the seedlings, hoping they would stick permanently.

Not only was it the coldest winter in memory the fact is they feared they would never survive that first winter. Sadly, some things are aborted before they start. Just as Roe vs. Wade. With a kerosene lamp in hand they got in a fetal position and worked well into the night on their mission. You have heard of "whistle while you work" this band of brothers prayed (literally) that the seedlings would not only survive but thrive!

As some time passed, I am certain that a few of the assistants complained that the work was too hard, the odds stacked against them, it's just another goodwill gift from another nation, who will ever recognize our efforts or realize if we stop now? Perhaps they thought the task was too difficult and since the gift was so small it wasn't worth their effort and sacrifice. While some may have slacked or cowered back, William Easton knew the fact that they were commissioned to do a job and do it well.

They plowed ahead and planted down despite the cold and rain and continued to plant while praying that the seeds would stick. This went on for days, weeks, months and miraculously their worked paid off. The seedlings survived the cold, sprouted and in time began to flourish! The National Park Service note at a public ceremony on March 27, 1912, First Lady Helen Taft and Viscountess Chinda, wife of the Japanese Ambassador planted two trees around the north bank of the Tidal Basin in West Potomac Park. Today, those two trees still stand tall at the terminus of 17th Street SW, marked by a large plaque. By 1915, the U.S. government responded with a gift of Dogwood trees to the people of Japan.

Ironically, this was not the first time this gesture of goodwill was to be planted in the minds and soil of America. A Japanese chemist named Jokichi Takamine happened to be in Washington, D.C. with the Honorable Midzuno, Japanese Consul to New York City on April 8, 1910. When informed of a petition to plant Japanese trees along the Speedway, Takamine asked the First Lady (Mrs. Taft) if she would accept two thousand trees, while Midzuno suggested that the trees be given in the name of "Tokyo." They finally had a meeting with the First Lady and she accepted the trees.

On April 13, 2010, Spencer Cosby whom was Superintendent of the Office of Public Buildings and Grounds purchased an additional ninety trees that were to be planted along the Potomac River stretching south from East Potomac Park to the north nestled around the Lincoln Memorial.

Things were progressing but then came to a halt. On August 30, the

Embassy of Japan in Washington, DC informed the U.S. Department of State that the city of Tokyo intended to donate two thousand plus trees to the United States to be planted along the Potomac. When the trees arrived an inspection performed by the Department of Agriculture revealed the trees were infected with insects and would have to be destroyed to protect local growers.

So close but so far away, President Taft gave the order to have the trees burned on January 28, 1910. Secretary of State Philander C. Knox wrote a letter of regret to the Japanese Ambassador. Takamine graciously responded quickly with the promise of additional trees, actually 3,020 in all, of a lineage swiped from a famous batch of trees along the Arakawa River. On February 14, 1912 all three thousand trees were shipped on board the Awa Maru and arrived in our Nation's Capital via train from Seattle on March 26, 1912.

Perseverance pays off because that big gesture between two countries and those small seedlings and the sacrifice of both blue and white collar servants helped the now renowned Cherry Blossoms take root in the heart of our American fabric and soil. We learn some valuable nuggets in this chapter. For starters, just because it isn't easy doesn't mean it can't be done. Secondly, the harder the obstacles, the greater the reward; and just because it starts off slowly, it doesn't mean it won't blossom to something spectacular!

The first Cherry Blossom Festival was held in 1935 under joint sponsorship by various groups and today is an annual event. The cherry trees had quickly become an established part of Washington, D.C. In 1938, plans to cut down some of the trees to clear valuable space around the Jefferson Memorial prompted a group of women to chain themselves together at the site in protest. As some men sat out, these women stood up and a compromise was reached where more trees would be planted along the south side of the Basin to frame in the Memorial. In 1940, the Cherry Blossom was conceived as a result of those famous trees.

On December 11, 1941, four trees were cut down. It has been suspected for decades that it was in direct retaliation for the attack on Pearl Harbor by the Empire of Japan four days earlier, though it could never be confirmed. In hopes of downplaying the scenario and hoping further attacks on the trees wouldn't take place, they were referred to as "Oriental" flowering trees for the duration of World War II. The Cherry Blossom Festivals were suspended during WWII, the Cherry Blossoms Festival resumed in 1947 with full support of the Washington, D.C. Board of Trade and Commissioners.

The following year (1948), the Japanese ambassador gave a 300 year old lantern made of stone to the City of Washington, D.C. commemorating the signing of 1854 Japan-US Treaty of Amity and Friendship by Commodore Matthew C. Perry. For several years, the lighting of that lantern formally opened the Cherry Festival. Three years later, the president of the pearl company founded by Mikimoto Kokichi donated the Mikimoto Pearl Crown. It contained more than 1,585 pearls and over five thousand pounds of pure gold! Today, the crown is still used at the coronation of the Festival Queen at the Grand Ball.

Japan graciously gave 3,800 additional Yoshino trees in 1965, which were given by First Lady "Lady Bird" Johnson in 1965. These trees specifically were planted on the grounds of the Washington Monument. For this occasion, the First Lady and Ryuji Takeuchi, wife of the Japanese ambassador, reenacted the 1912 planting.

Exactly a century later the trees are alive and more revered than ever before. Nearly one million tourists descend upon Washington, D.C. annually to admire and appreciate the beauty of the Cherry Blossoms. A celebration takes place for two weeks every year on the last Saturday of March to the second week of April. Endless exhibits abound for folks from around the globe and fun for all ages.

From the initial gift of 12 varieties of the 3,020 trees, the two that are most popular are the Yoshino and Kwanzan. The Yoshino produces a single, white blossom that creates an effect of white clouds around the Tidal Basin and north onto the grounds of the Washington Monument. Intermingled among them are Akebono cherry trees which blossom at the same time as the Yoshino and produce single, pink blossoms. The Kwanzan grows primarily in East Potomac Park and comes into bloom two weeks after the Yoshino. It produces clusters of clear, pink double blossoms and together with the National Mall as a backdrop are drop dead gorgeous. Yes, those seeds seemed small but God threw a "Cherry" on top!

Years ago, I heard of two masons who were laying brick. A pedestrian walking came across the first brick layer and inquired what he was building? The first responded with a smile, "I'm building a Cathedral, a modern day masterpiece!" The mason continued to work and the pedestrian walked on and at the end of the block saw the mason's colleague and asked him the same question. The other mason barked "Nothing special, just another building and a boring day at the office!" Here we find two men helping construct the same edifice and note the difference in attitude. The fact is almost all work is noble but our actions and attitude determine if we are going to help make history or be forgotten.

When William Easton and his team first got the call to plant a tree did they have a clue that their labors would result in something so monumental? What appeared as something so small and insignificant at the start, blossomed to something mighty at the end. The Bible says: "*Don't despise the day of small beginnings.*" When Easton and his team held the small seedlings in their hands, did they realize then they were "carrying greatness?" Did they press on and plant down because it had value or because they were honored to work and found work honorable? Was it the seedlings in their hand, the gift from a nation or their personal character that drove them to do a job well done, regardless if it were big or small? Perhaps all three are examples of greatness and the price of professionalism and class.

The name William Easton is most likely unfamiliar to you, but he is family to me!

William Easton, the head gardener of the U.S. Park Service in 1912, was born and raised in the Georgetown neighborhood of Washington, D.C. He is my maternal great-great-grandfather. Without a doubt, I cannot help but think that when he was planting the Cherry Blossoms he knew he was carrying greatness!

My mother, Sharon Lee Shelton found this newspaper clipping decades ago on my ancestor. He died when he was 78 years old on February 4, 1946. Netta Craig Turkenton wrote "St. Francis of Georgetown: A Memoir of Olde Georgetown."

"A saint has lived in our midst and he passed on to his reward, leaving in old Georgetown such a train of mourners as would glorify the memory of a great religious of Holy Church. ALL LOVED HIM. High and low estate, white and colored, young and old all loved this good man and paid their tribute of tears unrestrainedly at his passing. The very birds of the air and pigeons of the neighborhood lined up at attention on the rooftops adjacent to his home at the time of his death and one poor cat whose injuries he had healed and whom he fed daily, sat in gravest dignity before the door of his friend, a faithful watcher during that sad day, never learning his past. This man loved his fellows and his "little brethren" with the quality of tender compassion we ascribe to the gentle Nazarene Himself. Never known to speak ill of anyone, he was ever ready to cheer the hopeless, comfort the sorrowing, aid the needy. Especially was he tender with the young and aged.

They called him St. Francis II for he was the most often to be seen with his black spaniel, a large tortoise shell cat and many birds and pigeons – all crowding close about him seeking the ministrations of his kindly hands. Often on the fringe of the group were other animals awaiting his call to come closer. To see his loving care of all animals and his feeding of the poor starrelings of the harsh winter months was an experience never to be forgotten. These were pictures worthy of reproduction by some master artist. How very happy were we to receive with the smaller recipients of his love, his cheery smile, lifting word of greeting, a bit of advice about our own pets or with a quiet chat about some civic interest. We went out of our way many times for those things.

TENDED CHERRY TREES. This very gentle man attained his majority as he said, through his work as gardner-foreman for the East Potomac Park and the Department of Public Parks and Buildings. Here he befriended many abandoned pets and strays roaming at large and fed starving birds in winter seasons. And here under his loving supervision the famous Cherry Trees were planted and brought to their beautiful maturity after many hours of labor, prayers and unbreakable faith. When some years ago there was a cry against them, this devoted man felt that the slaughter of the innocents was imminent, his children imperiled. It was a dark period for him. When, however, truth and beauty prevailed again he was radiantly happy. REMEMBERED This

Spring, about Easter Sunday, the time of the Resurrection, we look to the Cherry Blossoms to show forth their glory. Here indeed Mr. William Easton of Georgetown, our St. Francis II has his beautiful memorial as well as in the hearts of his many friends of his community. When you look at the beauty of Washington, especially in Cherry Blossom time, you might remember: Mr. William Easton of Georgetown."

CHAPTER TWO

A CUP OF JOE

Meet Joe. His legal name was Joseph and this brother from another mother was not the first person in history, nor would he be the last, where others tried to "keep a good man down." Instead of helping a brother out, Joe's siblings beat him, sold him and left him for dead. They even tried to bury him alive. Appropriate because jealousy is crueler than the grave. Instead of grace he got grief!

In the book of Genesis, we meet a boy who by his actions was the man of his house. He may have been the runt of the pack but he was royalty in pursuit. Joseph was the eleventh of Jacob's twelve sons. His mother was Rachel and he was a son of Israel. He lived in Canaan with ten half-brothers, one full brother and one half-sister. He was the apple of his daddy's eye and in a land of nightmares at night he was a dreamer by day.

It is not the bad dreams at night that scare others away. It is those who have the audacity to dream by day and actually accomplish them along the way! Very few notice when we dream at night but almost everyone watches when dreams become reality in broad daylight. It has been said: "Most people want you to do well just not real well." However, you should never become less for someone to love you more. If they cannot handle you at your best, then perhaps they should become one of the rest-- content with mediocrity and not genuine ministry.

Joseph was the man! He was athletic, handsome and blessed by God with many gifts and talents. He was smart and blessed beyond measure socially. He was confident, captivating and charismatic. He had charm and also character.

Joseph would tell us today that integrity will drive us further down the road of life than the automobile "Infiniti." He was hard working and good looking. With his powerful attributes, even thousands of years ago, he was on a roll!

His father lavished him with love and in his eye, Joseph could do nothing wrong. Joseph was a man on the move and the only thing in his way was the insecurity of the brothers around him. Joseph's father gave him a jacket. A coat of many colors and it was expensive and extravagant. It drew attention to both the giver of the gift and recipient of the garment. Just like Joseph, the coat had substance, style and sizzle. When he walked, others talked and some balked. Some said what was already true: "Joseph is on a roll! He's going places!! Did you see that coat his father gave him? While some saw him as being on a roll, most began to roll their eyes with both anger and resentment.

Rather than compliment, they complained; but it didn't stop there. They began to secretly plot how they could not only demote him but also derail and destroy him. JeaLOUSY is plain lousy. We all lose when we cannot appreciate the blessings and good fortune of another.

PRIDE is what banned Satan out of Heaven and it goes before every fall. It is no accident that the middle letter in "pride" and "sin" is I. Ironically, pride and promotion can cause trouble for us all if we are not careful. Pride may hinder you from getting a promotion or another's pride may try to cease you from getting it or acquiring it for very long. It was the pride of his brothers that caused them to go wild with envy and their behavior was out of control. Rather than rejoicing with those who rejoice, and weeping with those who weep, they began to work. Not to work hard at advancing their own dreams but at dashing Joseph's dreams.

Their private pain and now exposed public pride against their brother turned into an all out plot to replace his dreams with a nightmare of his own. They did the unthinkable and contemplated killing him. The Bible says "nothing new under the sun." They went from harassing him to hurting him and then holding him captive. They threw him in a cistern and considered leaving him for dead.

It is ironic, he was thrown in a well because they thought "Oh, well!" Once he is out of sight – he's out of mind! So they thought -- but guilt is a heavy weight to carry and just because one isn't around doesn't mean you can get them off your mind. It is a guilty conscience that creeps into your mental rear view mirror with relentless pursuit and if you don't pull over and repent it will run you down!

The eldest brother, Reuben didn't want Joseph to die. He could have been the first "Reuben Sandwich" because he was stuck between his brothers' bologna and Joseph was the big cheese! It is fitting that the cheese on a Reuben sandwich is Swiss because their plan had holes all in it. Personally, he really didn't want any part of his siblings' sinister plan. Initially, Reuben intended to rescue his brother and return him to his father; but like most failed robbery attempts, the perfect crime doesn't always go according to plan. Interesting that when Joseph's brothers first apprehended him the very first thing they did was to strip him of his prized possession. They tore off the coat that his Daddy had given him because they despised the individual (Joseph) but also hated his identity. His coat was an outward expression of his inner drive.

Satan in the Garden also attacked Adam and Eve's identity. He made them doubt who they were, where they were and who God is. If the enemy or your "friends" can cause you to doubt your worth, then it is quite possible you are on a slippery slope, too. The reason they despised Joseph was not the colorful coat but the colossal call of God on his life. They had a career but he had a calling. They were stuck in the now but Joseph had a future as bright as the desert sun. He was going places and they were stuck in reverse and it drove Joseph's brothers' nuts!

What they failed to see was you may strip the cloak or coat but you cannot take away the call of God. Read that again, because that will flat out preach! They are irrevocable and woven together. Phil Collins had an album "No Jacket Required" and Joseph knew it was necessary to wear the jacket now to see success with Jesus in the future. He was appointed by his earthly father to wear the coat, but anointed by his Heavenly Father with the call to carry out the plan He had for him. Take comfort in knowing that you may get knocked down, picked over and left for dead but if God be for you WHO can be against you?

While Joseph was licking his wounds and trying to learn what was right side up while upside down, things appeared to get worse. His brothers saw a caravan of camels coming to town and some Ishmaelites en route selling merchandise. Still not certain of their plan with what to do with Joseph, the older brother, Judah who was also the strongest, elected not to kill him but "sell" him. They bartered their brother, sold their sibling and auctioned off their very own for twenty pieces of silver. You don't need a Judas when you got a Judah. Call it inflation, but Joseph was sold for about the same price of Jesus years later.

After selling out, rather than stepping up as men, they now had to go back and cover their tracks. You cannot move forward backsliding as a believer. Similar to Jack Nicholson in the snow in the 1980 movie "The Shining" they both tried to cover up their sins (tracks) so guilt didn't point to them. Coming from a fifth generation Washington, D.C. law enforcement family, it has been said "the guilty always return to the scene of the crime."

They had already confiscated the coat of colors and now damaged it more with the blood of a goat. They made up an alibi to tell their aging and nearly blind father that his beloved son had been killed. They lied, saying Joseph had died, and tried horribly to weep as if they were sad. When you are mad, it is hard to be sad; but they could have won an Academy Award for best supporting actors mourning the death of the star of this drama, Joseph.

Another thing I have learned is you cannot count out the man that Satan couldn't knock out. Just because you are down doesn't mean that God is done. The brothers, despite being dumb, displayed wise theology because the goat's blood resembled Joseph's death as symbolic of the future blood of God that would keep him, sustain him and deliver him. The blood of Jesus would be more than sufficient in advance for the life of Joseph regardless if in a pit or palace.

What others meant for evil, God always means for good. We serve a good God! Their pride became Joseph's PROMOTION. Only God could write this script and Joseph was sold to serve Potiphar, the captain of Pharaoh's guard. Joseph found favor with God above and man below and was promoted to be his personal assistant. Joseph had some Major League helpers but minor league haters. Sadly, sometimes a prophet is respected everywhere but home.

Had Joseph not had endured going down he would have never appreciated going up. He had to be rejected so he could accept his new duties and serve with honor yet humility. Joseph was eventually assigned to oversee Potiphar's entire household as superintendent.

Joseph was criticized, not for being incompetent, but because he was too competent. Girls wanted to date him and unless men were comfortable in their own skin they acted as if he didn't exist or worse, wanted him dead. However, the Bible is clear: "a righteous man may fall seven times and rise again, but the wicked shall fall by calamity (Proverbs 24:16)." Joseph was handsome as a boy but gorgeous as a man. Just because you honor God doesn't mean you are not a man! Anyone can be a boy but it takes grace and guts to be a man of God. When you are God's man you are nobody's boy! Joseph, still sore from the private rejection of his brothers, is now appreciating the newfound responsibilities publicly serving in leadership. The problem with leadership is it is lovely but can be lonely.

Having been rejected by his family, the reward of a bigger resume among royalty could have been a recipe for disaster with what was coming around the corner. The very wife of the man who loved him like a son and entrusted him with power is now on the prowl and has Joseph in her sights. She was a 'cougar' and a 'Desperate Housewife' rolled into one. She not only had power but also time on her hands and looks that would make most men get weak. Joseph could have easily looked for love in all the wrong places. He could have gotten arrogant and believed his own press clippings and even felt entitled to be with this accommodating woman. He was entrusted to serve his master's wealth and empire. Why not add the attractive wife of his boss into the mix? It was tempting and his for the taking. Potiphar was slowing down sexually and his wife was warming up. Who would know of this love affair?

In the moment of intense temptation too often we think we have to look graceful getting out of town. Wrong! Better to look foolish fleeing from sin than look elegant falling smack into it. Sometimes you don't get blessed for staying, but for running! She was hot, he was in heat and something was going to happen in a hurry. He had a dilemma. Was he going to live by faith or succumb to the flesh? He elected to honor his earthly boss and

Heavenly Father not dishonor. You cannot honor the Son and delve into sin simultaneously.

She was willing and fortunately he wasn't and like Elvis, he left the building and ran out of the bedroom faster than a future Ferrari. However, before he was gone, she reached for his cloak and grabbed it. It was a coat that got him in trouble the first time and darn if it isn't his cloak that tried to trap him this time. It has been said, "Hell hath no fury like the scorn of a woman." He left but since she didn't get what she wanted, with evidence in hand, she thought she had him RIGHT where she wanted. His brothers wanted him *dead*, she wanted him in *bed* but this *led* straight to God's plan.

Just like before, the enemy (Accuser of the Brethren) went after his identity and integrity. If he was dead his brothers could move on and if he was out of mind then her conscience could be cleared to ease her sin and his resentment of the attractive offer of adultery. Sin is attractive at the start but profoundly ugly in the middle and end.

Their pride and God's promotion now set the stage for Joseph's PRISON.

How can one do right and be treated so wrong? This was not only bad but royally bad! About this juncture almost anyone or everyone would consider their Christianity. Keep in mind that Christianity is not a religion but relationship and not built on our emotions but His devotion to us. Feelings are fickle but faith is forever. It is one thing to take pain and setback when we have done wrong but it's hard to wrap our head and hearts around when bad things happen to good people.

Joseph knew that honoring God was the promotion. Regardless, if in a palace or prison the privilege of knowing Him and making Him known was worth all the gold in Egypt. Don't miss this because this is good. Actually God! The brothers took his *coat*, Potiphar's wife took his *cloak,* but neither of them could take what mattered most: God's *call* on Joseph's life and his complete faith in the Almighty! Keep in mind, that God's call on your life and His gifts to you are without repentance (Romans 11:29). Today, they may take your coat, cars, cash, college degree, court side seats or country club membership but Christ cannot be extracted from our lives. It is not so much us holding on to Him as He holding us.

We now find Joseph in an all too familiar scenario. He is imprisoned and he has his back against the wall. It has been said "How you act at your lowest point reveals who you really are." Better to be demoted for doing right than promoted for doing wrong. My mom said something to me as a child that has assisted me well into adulthood: "Frankie, better to make the last page of the paper for doing right than make front page news for doing wrong." Sometimes no news is Good News!

In prison you have time to think. First of all you will learn quickly who you really are. Secondly, you learn who your real friends are and most importantly, learn who God is. The Lord never changes and friends may flee and family may fail but God sticks closer than a brother! Christ is a companion that never leaves and concrete bars and isolation cannot separate you from the love of Jesus.

Interesting enough that outside of his father's respect, Joseph never found favor with his brothers; however, outsiders saw his value. Honestly, it's not that they didn't see it but they were too envious to see the obvious. Most folks would rather stay small than compliment others in a big way. Since their dream is small they want to criticize, choke and even consider killing you so they can exist but still never live.

Joseph was rejected at home but promoted abroad. He was promoted in the palace and once again promoted but now is in prison. His brothers tried, but Joseph is living proof you cannot keep a good man down. He was placed in charge of the prisoners by the warden. He was a leader in both camps and God orchestrated events and strategically placed some friends in prison with him. Joseph reunites with Pharaoh's chief cup-bearer and baker in prison. The two employees of his former boss had dreams and Joseph offered to interpret them on one condition -- that they would not forget him and assist with his release from prison.

We learn two traits here: Joseph interpreted dreams because he had a God given gift. He did it on the mountain or in the valley. He did it when he felt like it or even while contemplating quitting. When you have a gift you cannot just turn it on or off. You cannot serve the Lord based on emotion but on devotion. Secondly, he knew his gift was to not only honor God but also to help others regardless if it was reciprocated or not. Joseph gave liberty to others with unlocking their prison (literally) but he was left shackled sitting out and still stuck. Society is quick to ask for help but slow to say thanks. They got reinstated but he was reduced to sitting on the inside looking out.

Eventually, the cup-bearer did remember Joseph and spoke of his skill to Pharaoh and Joseph was eventually released from prison. The Pharaoh took off his personal signet ring and placed it on Joseph's finger, clothed him in fine linens and put a gold necklace around his neck. Had Joseph never encountered private pain he wouldn't be worthy to wear public praise. If that wasn't enough, he went from the pit to the palace and a prison before coming second to Pharaoh. He endured problems before the promotion and now the Prime Minister made him king at thirty years old, he was one of most powerful men in the world. Looking back what was a demotion in the natural was a promotion in the Spiritual.

His brothers' pride and God's promotion gave him the PROMISE he always longed for. His goal was to never outdo his siblings but love and be loved by them. Even when the reunion took place after a great famine in the land he could have destroyed them, belittled them or worse, act like they didn't exist. He was the bigger man at the beginning and the mature man at the end. What every man longs for is respect and in this case he got the two things he desperately desired most: respect and reconciliation.

Nelson Mandela had many great quotes but one of them Joseph with the coat of many colors could really relate to and all of us can learn from. The late African president said, "There is no passion to be found playing small in settling for a life that is less than the one you are capable of living." Yes, Mandela had a less than perfect past but then again we all have and he learned valuable lessons while incarcerated, paid for his mistakes and was transformed into a better man and great leader. President Bill Clinton went to South Africa and visited Mandela in the same prison where he spent nearly three decades of his life in jail. The current United States President asked the former South African president if he wanted to knock some heads when they finally set him free. Mandela in his trademark smile replied, "When I first left that prison I wanted to let them have it for how they mistreated me but

I realized I had to forgive them even if they never asked for it. The fact is, if I harbored any hatred towards those who hurt me I would be still shackled in my mind despite walking out a free man." Powerful! One attribute of carrying greatness is also willing to forgive. Proper political protocol dictates that the first few rows of an inauguration are reserved for dignitaries and heads of state. Mandela did the unthinkable and in lieu of placing prominent politicians in the front of his swearing in for his presidency he placed the same prison guards who mistreated him, hurt him and spat on him. He was symbolically and subliminally stating two things simultaneously. One, the past is the past and forgiveness is powerful. Secondly, as he spoke behind the presidential podium with those men in the front rows he was also relaying a message 'don't forget who is in charge now."

Joseph showed great compassion and class with his brothers. He could have destroyed them but what they meant for evil God used for his good. I am convinced that they will still have to give an account for their actions but Joseph was not only vindicated but became a better man in the process. My college friend, Clayton King is teaching pastor at NewSpring Church in Anderson, SC and campus minister at Liberty University in Lynchburg, VA. We have been friends exactly for twenty years (January 1994)! He has said for decades that there is nothing like a hot cup of coffee on a cold fall morning. Over the years, I always had cream and sugar in my coffee but Clayton loves his black. Lately, because of my admiration and friendship for him I gave up on the cream and today drink it dark too. One of my favorite books in the Bible is Hebrews. Remember that God's involvement in our lives resembles making coffee; we can take great comfort that "He Brews." Coffee beans are grinded and that is how we get coffee grounds. Keep in mind with God constantly present (regardless if in a prison or promotion) we are standing on "holy ground."

Today, it makes no difference what season you are in as you read this book may this cup of Joe (Joseph) bring you a fresh fire and focus that comes from one of the world's greatest ambassadors of patriotism and perseverance. He was knocked down but definitely not out and the coat he adored and adorned was great but it was the call of God on his life that carried him through the good, bad and ugly. He got through it and you will too!

In closing with a cup of Joe I will leave you with a bowl of blessing. Friends, you will never get ahead if you live to get even. It is a cancer with no remission and a dead end street. Approximately fifteen years ago while working full-time on Capitol Hill in politics I was also a part-time minister of youth in Maryland. A large Christian event called "Acquire the Fire" was coming to Baltimore, and I took two 15- passenger vans filled with teens to the convention center where nearly 10,000 were present. The place was packed and the speaker came out. He was 6'7 tall but I was sitting nearly three rows from the top and despite looking small on stage he was larger than life on the jumbo screen. He was absolutely brilliant and brought the house down. Half way through his message I remember being so inspired that I felt God leading me to transition as an itinerant speaker. Not to be seen but believing that God deposited seeds of greatness in me and it was a message He wanted others to hear.

I trusted Christ as my Lord and Savior at age seven but I remember vividly that night I wanted to walk from the top of the nosebleeds (seats) all the way to the front not to "get saved" but shake the hand of the speaker to say thank you. His message blessed me immeasurably. Before the program started I had met another youth minister from another church when we first got settled in our seats. After his message and during intermission I leaned over to ask the youth pastor what he thought of that sermon we just heard. I will never forget his expression or response. He couldn't compliment him to save his own life, he rolled his eyes and as if his tongue didn't come through customs snarled and said sarcastically: "I guess he was all right but didn't do much for me." My heart dropped and then I realized that he was too small to compliment what God chose to do "big" in another person's life. Two wrongs don't make a right so I allowed him to his wrong opinion and gathered my youth group and started the trek back outside in the cold to our two awaiting vans.

While walking to our vans, the Lord impressed on me to ask Sam Glenn to be the speaker at our upcoming Youth Rally scheduled the following year. I just knew that he would be super for our outreach and couldn't wait to tell my youth group. We got them accounted for and as they got in the vans I got on the CB radio we had and was thrilled to share with them the good news that the speaker who just brought the house down may be our speaker in the future. When I relayed the message to both our van and the one next to us under the sound of my voice via radio the response was not what I expected. Actually, it was the same awkward silence resembling the jealous youth pastor I just left in the convention center.

How could this be? Am I oblivious to something or like my opening statement in this book the obvious isn't obvious. You could hear a pin drop and the silence was deafening. I was hoping for my crowd to cheer but a choir of crickets was all you could hear! They were not jealous but I learned that at that moment they hadn't heard directly from Jesus. One of my students sheepishly spoke up and said: "Pastor Frank, it's not that we didn't like him because he was AMAZING but we can't see why a guy who just spoke to ten thousand would actually come to our little church? Their reply was sincere but I was crushed. God had already told me to contact Sam Glenn's office the next week and try to learn what it would take to bring him back to our church and now my own team (youth group) was telling me to not even try. Why bother?

If you are not careful you can let those closest to you make you miss your moment. They can talk you out of the dream that God deposited in you and the four worse words in Webster's Dictionary strewn together are "What Might Have Been?" Dr. Johnny Hunt said, "If you can't see it before you see it you will never see it." How true! I submit to you that if you don't see it before others see it neither of you will see it. God will give you the vision and you may have to walk alone to the victory. The key is don't lose heart.

It was a long ride back to church that night. We just had a mountain top high but their remarks made me feel so low. God said invite and that was all I could think of that night. You have two options in life you hear the loud critics or still small voice of Christ. We arrived at church and I did my best to not let them know they hurt me and hugged and high fived them goodnight as they dashed to their respective rides home. As I drove back home in the dark, I remembered the instruction from The Light. Monday morning arrived and I knew Sam's hometown of Chicago was an hour behind and I stared at the phone just waiting to call his office at 9 AM their time to try to see if he would come. My mind was saying "no" my own youth group said "no" and the jealous theologian from the other church that night was adamant his opinion was "no" too.

What was it going to be? Just sit back and do nothing or risk trying even if it wasn't meant to be? I called and his secretary was super kind and we discussed our intentions and learned his fee and would he come speak at our youth rally? Truthfully, Sam didn't come once. Actually, he came TWO years in a row and at the time ours was the largest youth rally of its kind in our region and God showed up! Long story short, Sam and I became great friends. Lesson number one – who you respect is who you attract.

Sam became a mentor to me and asked me to be Vice President of his National Christian Youth Speakers Network along with Miss Colorado and Miss Missouri. We wrote five books together and would you believe he was the "Best Man" in my wedding and then he flew me to Chicago, Illinois to officiate his wedding! Twice he asked me to join him and speak on his stage in front of 7,000 teens with Rebecca St. James and David Nasser. We saw over 500 teens publicly repent of sin and trust Christ by faith and when they came out of their seats and ran down those bleachers it sounded like rain on a tin roof and music to my ears! That night I was on the big screen speaking and would have missed it all if I had let envy, jealousy and the lack of vision of those around me be my guide. Truth be told, today by God's grace and a faith of a mustard seed, we have now been in 48 states, over a dozen countries and preached on world-wide television and tapped International Evangelism Chairman of 2012 Olympics outreach in London, England with Lay Witnesses For Christ.

Jealousy will keep you grounded but faith and honor will help you soar to astronomical heights. If I had listened to the critics or the crowd, I would have missed what Christ designed and destined for me. Others are still sitting in the nosebleeds but God blessed to be on the stage, not because I needed to be seen, but knew I was carrying greatness and God's message needed to be heard. It is costly to be jealous and a jerk but it pays to resemble Jesus. You can sit and sulk in the shadows sitting down or you can trust God, dig deep and stand up and graduate from mediocrity to true ministry. You will either carry greatness or bury greatness but you can't do both. The clock is ticking, time is wasting and the world is waiting. Get up because anyone can sit out.

CHAPTER THREE

"MARY, I KNOW YOU KNEW"

In the first century we come across two women. One named Elisabeth and the other Mary. One was dying to conceive and for the other would you believe pregnancy was not on her radar. Elisabeth was too old and Mary was too young. Elisabeth was married, unsuccessful with her man and couldn't and Mary never tried and did! Elisabeth attempted for decades to get pregnant and struck out. Mary wasn't even married and never intimate with a man and with some Holy Help hit a grand slam and gave birth to the Son of Man.

Both loved God and honored Him. Both had felt rejected and knew the pain to live like outcasts. Both were not famous but were found to be faithful. Ironically, both birthed boys with names beginning with "J." Elisabeth bore John and Mary birthed Jesus. What was impossible for man was possible with God.

Elisabeth was the daughter of Aaron, the high priest. She was married to Zacharias and they were model citizens. Elisabeth loved God and was born into prestige and prominence. Mary, on the other hand, was an Israelite Jew from Nazareth in Galilee. She didn't know power but poverty. She had no wealth, no fame and we still don't know her last name! She was a virgin and it's fitting that God would pick these two women totally different but united in love with God and life.

When you feel as if the parade has passed you by one never takes things for granted when better days come to town. Elisabeth was despised because she couldn't reproduce. It was her dream to raise a child and love them with her whole being. It wasn't that she wasn't worthy but God up to that time didn't allow things to work according to her plan. God is never in a hurry but always on time. God was not punishing her but preparing her for a task greater than she could imagine. However, preparation comes before promotion even in the dictionary. Elisabeth not only felt dejected but probably better off dead in that dark, dry season in her life. Family talked behind her back, friends began to distance themselves from her and she felt inadequate and incomplete.

She was isolated, grew depressed and felt as if hope was available to everyone but her. She became secluded and learned that although friends flee and family can be fickle that God the Father was faithful and never failed. Up to that point Elisabeth had been sidelined. Not just in public, but privately, and she felt excluded from the Major League of Motherhood deduced to playing on some minor league farm team never to return with the privilege of pregnancy and parenting.

If one is not careful we can get envious, jealous and hateful when bundles of blessings fall into the lap of others. Today, a woman who played by the rules and tried repeatedly to get pregnant could get really offended when a teenager not even married gets pregnant! Especially, two thousand years ago when teenage pregnancy was unheard of! It would be easy to get pious in a predicament like this. Everyone wants to throw rocks but the Babe yet to be birthed in her cousin's womb would in time become the Chief Cornerstone. Trying times are not only tough but can stretch us when it appears that everyone is blessed but us.

Elisabeth realized that two wrongs don't make a right and you cannot promote low living if you want to honor the Most High God. By God's grace and faithfulness, both in time became pregnant and their two baby boys would change the world. Talk about "Boys to Men" this dynamic duo were the originals! However, like all pregnancies, labor would come before the delivery. Elisabeth was ridiculed because she couldn't produce and Mary was almost killed because she got pregnant prematurely. It's difficult in any time of history to tell your significant other that you are pregnant but it's not because of you!

That line would break up a relationship almost 100% of the time. What do you mean you are pregnant? You want to marry me when you have been intimate with someone else?? If the relationship is this bad before the wedding what good can happen after the marriage??? Two thousand years ago, Joseph probably thought: "Mary, so let me get this straight. We are not married. YOU are pregnant and it's not my child and I am supposed to believe that God in Heaven is the Father?" You can almost picture Arnold (Gary Coleman) of the 1980's television sitcom, "Diff'rent Strokes" looking at his older brother with his trademark reply, "What you talking about Willis??"

For a man who didn't drink he may have been tempted to throw one down after hearing that alibi from his girl, but the Bible notes that Joseph was an honorable man, feared God and lived right. He was a bud who was wiser for his faith therefore didn't need Budweiser. Mark this down, you don't need the "king of beers" when your woman is carrying the King of kings! Joseph had faith in God and in his woman and yes, the child growing within her would enable him to be the step father of the Child who would mature into more than a man but the Messiah leading us up 'by faith' to the stairway of Heaven.

Just because Joseph was on board and Jesus was in her belly, it didn't mean that everyone else in their hometown was thrilled with this news. To them it was bad news but little did they know she was carrying GOOD NEWS. Mother Mary was the first to carry the Gospel. The crowd didn't realize it but she was carrying more than Good News but greatness and God all at once. When you dedicate your life and gifts to the Lord then you are intertwined with the Trinity and a three cord rope is impossible to break.

No one was happy for Mary and Joseph nor were they waiting in line to congratulate them or planning a baby shower. In that day, women actually married before conceiving babies. Here is a word for someone. What others see as illegitimate God sees legitimate to use to show grace to another and glory to Him. Just because others want to throw you out, God is calling you in and getting ready to promote you up! The crowd was sincere but sincerely wrong. Just like many today still miss Jesus they misjudged His mother, too. They rejected Mary, disrespected and borderline harassed her. The irony is they judged her but had no clue that the baby she bore (outside of grace) would judge them.

Mary heard the news when Elisabeth was six months pregnant. She was thrilled for her older relative and celebrated the fact. In life, I have found the greats are gracious and outside of Christ that pain is the common denominator. Both women went through tough times, baseless accusations, unfair resentment and a period of isolation. They were both exiled and seemed to be demoted before the uncertain promotion. They knew all too well what it was like to be considered trash yet were holding treasures. They were on the sidelines as pregnant mothers but boy their babes would win the game in life. They were not on "injured reserves" but I'm certain their feelings were injured and their emotional reserves were running low. Elisabeth and Mary while pregnant knew what it was like to be alone in the wilderness but both would tell us today with tears of joy two things: "God is faithful and don't waste your wilderness."

God prepared them in private before they were pregnant in public. Not everyone you meet is mature enough to babysit your baby but keep in mind they won't all throw a party for your dreams either. These women "carrying greatness" with bundles of boys and JOY would tell you as well as Joseph from previous chapter that they would prefer to plan your funeral. God doesn't entrust everyone with producing the same exact blessing and the favor of the Lord is not always fair. Leadership is lovely but also lonely but the price is worth the pain leading up to the birthing of God's miracle in you! We learn more in the incubator of God's adversity than the non-accredited school of Satan's lies and low living.

When we are in the wilderness we tend to hear from God more when the critics and crowds have been silenced. The noise of the world will try to drown out the still, small voice of the Lord. Your wilderness is not a demotion but a promotion that you failed to see. What was an obstacle at the start is your best opportunity for the rest of your life. Those who have been in the wilderness in private have an assignment to help others in public.

Those who are alone and hear from God in the closet will have something to say to mankind in the marketplace. Both Elisabeth and Mary were able to take their eyes off their critics and place them on the future Christ. Their trust in God carried them through and it will work the same for you!

The day that Mary went to visit Elisabeth picture this. Both women were pregnant with protruding bellies and when Mary walked in spoke and said "hi" to Elisabeth the Bible says clearly that the lad leapt, John jumped and the unborn boy bounced in his mother's womb. The reason John the future Baptist bounced and went bonkers is not just that Jesus was inches away in His mother's womb but that the God of the Universe was now in the same room!

In every courthouse across America each day before a case is tried regardless if one is a plaintiff or defendant, an attorney wearing a thousand dollar suit, a member of the jury or the janitor, you will always hear two words before the trial starts: "ALL RISE." Out of respect, everyone and I mean everyone, stands up for the one wearing the robe. I submit to you that the reason John jumped and stood up because when the Babe in the making was already The King of Kings for the taking and he couldn't help but rise in his mother's belly. One day, soon everyone will rise and then bow at the feet of The King wearing the Robe of Righteousness. This also shows the world that John was a child, not a choice, and although he wasn't seen he was very much alive! We should not abort babies! Adoption is greater than abortion. Don't let another abort the assignment God placed in you.

Just before Elisabeth gave birth to John the Bible notes Mary went home. Why did she leave? For one, she was still pregnant with Jesus. Secondly, when you are carrying God (Jesus) you don't have to wait around for good (John). To John's credit he knew Jesus before he was born and the blessing was he never got over Him! Read that again, have you ever considered that the two knew each other before they were born? It is interesting that when Elisabeth was in her wilderness before pregnancy that when she gave birth to John we read in Luke 1:82 that he was ushered out to his wilderness. Mary was in a wilderness after being beaten up verbally by callous people who were too blind to see the plan of the Lord and His will for her life. The irony is when Mary's wilderness stopped, her Son, Jesus' wilderness started immediately the first day of His ministry after being baptized by John.

Keep in mind, the next time you are feeling like you are in the wilderness it may not because you are bad but because God is good and He realizes you are carrying greatness. He is refining your character as He is defining your calling and your time away enables you to play your role with more fire and fervor later on the larger stage. Practice doesn't make perfect but persecution and pain do! Praise Him in your storm. Both Elisabeth and Mary would certainly be keynote speakers at future "Women of Faith" events. They knew faith, fear but favor all rolled into one and found their Heavenly Father faithful. Their test today became their TESTimony tomorrow!

When John was born he was exiled to the wilderness and we don't see him again until his public ministry as a man. I'm convinced that the day Jesus was born was when Christ crawled out of the crib and He was already crawling towards the cross. The Babe born in Bethlehem was birthed to die. Jesus taught us how to execute in life but our sins executed Him in death.

When the Wise Men came they brought expensive gifts to honor Jesus. They were wise not because they brought *gifts* but because they were willing to be in His *Presence*. They came from a great distance and carried earthly treasures but the kid who was already King would eventually carry them later in their lives.

John and Jesus shared a special bond. John knew Jesus intimately and he served Him faithfully throughout his life. When John came out of the wilderness after years in isolation and living in the wild, I am convinced most folks probably smelled him before they saw him. When you have been in the wilderness you tend to talk funny, walk funny, look funny and act funny but most certainly smell funny! Again, those who hear from God in private have something to say to others in public.

John probably resembled John Rambo and the entire cast of "Duck Dynasty." Place them all in a blender and what poured out was John the Baptist! He had faith and facial hair! That brother ate locusts and wild honey. His wardrobe was not the most fashionable made by man but he sure was faithful to God. At that moment, all eyes were on John. He was doing the Lord's work and literally waist deep in ministry as he baptized folks in the river. John is a great example of integrity because when you start out strong it is tempting to ease up or wander off before the finish. John promoted faith but could have slipped into the flesh.

If the disciples drove a Honda because "they were all in one Accord" than I believe John the Baptist could relate to a Toyota because the Bible tells us he was the "Forerunner" to Jesus! Once John left the wilderness of his youth he knew his mission as a man and produced. Sometimes in ministry we can be so busy doing the work of the Lord that we leave out the Lord of the work.

We find John baptizing and a crowd had gathered around. Four centuries had passed since a prophet preached with such power and now this wild man out of the wilderness had quite the following. In that moment, all eyes were on John and from the back of the crowd came Christ. Had John neglected his assignment, grabbed the glory of God and promoted himself more than Jesus, we could have had some serious problems. Without missing a beat, John knew that he had to decrease so He could increase and that he was born for this moment! John said with a shout, "Prepare ye the way of the Lord" and "Behold the Lamb of God who takes away the sin of the world." John promoted Jesus and Jesus promoted John by allowing him the high honor to baptize the God of Heaven with a crowd on Earth watching.

What I love about John is twofold. First, he knew his role. He was a messenger delivering the Messiah's mail. He was to point The Way but never pretended to be the answer. John lived and died sharing wherever, whenever and to whoever would listen that Christ is our only hope to Heaven. Today, he would have preached to presidents and prisoners, from Hollywood to homeless and to white collar, blue collar and those with "ring around the collar." He preached with power above and urgency below and saw scores come to saving faith in Christ. Secondly, I love that John never *got over God.*

Had both of their mothers not endured such personal pain these boys, now men, would not have been able to be such a corporate blessing. What looked like a lost cause was the exact recipe for salvation that God had planned all along. Had John tried to eclipse the Son and steal some of the credit, he would have been no better than Satan. Just because we start out strong doesn't mean we will finish well. John inspires me and encourages us all that he LEAPT before he was born when meeting Jesus; he LIVED for Him his entire life and LOVED the Lord even in death. John lost his head over Christ but never lost his heart. Deep inside, John knew that he was privileged to be part of God's plan but salvation was not found in anyone outside of Christ.

John the Baptist knew intimately these traits:

* John was good but Jesus is God.
* John was God's man but Jesus is God of Man
* John had a mission but Jesus is Messiah
* John had a message but Jesus is The Message
* John was one but Jesus is part of the Trinity yet all three in one
* John pointed the way but Jesus is The Way, Truth & Life (John 14:6)
* John was the forerunner but Jesus is the First and Last
* John baptized with water but Jesus baptized with fire
* John promoted Jesus and Jesus promoted John
* John died serving Jesus but Jesus died to save John and you!

In ministry, we can be guilty of giving ministers too much credit or not enough. Mother Mary and John were good but they were not God. It was grace that God would use them and amazing grace that He would use us. Jesus said: "No man born of woman was greater than John." What a compliment from the God of the Universe! God has a way of promoting those who promote Him. You may not get the accolades on Earth but will certainly be rewarded in Heaven.

John speaks to us today and above we learned "Who Was" John but he tells us with the same boldness today don't "Waste your Wilderness." Without a doubt, John was "Wild and pointed The Way." Frankly, John wasn't looking for followers on Twitter or friends on Facebook and could care less if you "liked" his page because he didn't care if you got him; all that consumed John was that you got Jesus! You can befriend a Christian and attend a church and be nice to clergy and still die without Christ. John wasn't promoting a religion but he was dying to give you a real relationship with the Redeemer.

He was not only wild and pointed the way but he was a "Warrior for the Word." The same Clayton that loves his coffee black shared a sermon once and closed with a story about Evangelist Charles Finney. It was reported that the fiery preacher was holding meetings just blocks from The White House in 1832. The President at that time was Andrew Jackson and one of his Cabinet members told the Commander- in- Chief, "Preacher Finney is in town and I believe it would be worth our while to hear what he has to say." In case you missed the memo, God is greater than government.

To President Jackson's credit, he agreed, and that night they walked (no motorcade) to attend the meeting where a capacity crowd had gathered to hear this itinerant preacher. Minutes before the service was to start, an assistant to Finney searched frantically for him but without success. For the life of him he could not find the famed preacher and with two minutes to spare he spotted him. The fiery preacher was in the dark and on the floor face down like a snake alone with his nose planted in an open Bible and was pleading with the God of the Universe for power from on high to minister to the assembled crowd. He was praying one more time in the dark to promote the Light.

Finney's aide got on his knees and whispered: "Preacher, you are on in a minute and we must go." The Evangelist responded: "Thank you" but he never moved. The slightly frustrated assistant noted: "By the way, the President of the United States is in the church house tonight to hear you speak." As if he didn't comprehend what he said and with his nose still buried in The Book he replied, "I appreciate that." Growing almost furious with each passing nanosecond, the assistant implored for the last time, "Preacher, we are supposed to be out there NOW and the most powerful man in the world is waiting on you to come out and preach!" Finney didn't budge and said, "Thank you."

The assistant left and right behind him was the preacher and he walked out and humbly placed his Bible on the pulpit. He looked at the standing room only crowd with folks literally hanging over the balcony with great expectancy. Finney searched the audience and opened with these words, "It has come to my attention that the President of the United States of America is present tonight." Then, he spotted President Jackson in the second row and without missing a beat, and with compassion in his heart and the authority of Heaven in his voice, said with tears looking directly at Jackson: "Mr. President, if you don't repent on the Lord Jesus Christ, sir you will split Hell wide open like anyone else without salvation."

The crowd was silent and others were speechless. How could one man speak with such power and boldness yet with humility and compassion all at once? Finney, like John the Baptist, knew true power was in God above not government below. Secondly, they didn't waste their wilderness and never wavered in their call or commitment to Christ. They were not looking to be seen but knew the story needed to be heard and because they promoted God the Creator promoted them!

Mark Lowry penned that Christmas classic "Mary Did You Know?" decades ago. Looking back two thousand years ago, millions pondered and cannot help but still wonder if Mary and Elisabeth knew they were carrying greatness. Initially, I wanted to name this chapter, "Mary, Did you Know?" Without question, I believe they did, and praise God that they, unlike their critics, didn't chase the big thing and miss the biggest gift of all. Elisabeth gave birth to the one who pointed the way and Mary delivered God who is the Way, Truth and Life. Mary, by God's grace delivered Jesus in birth, but Jesus, by His grace delivered her in His death.

My dear friend, Dr. Johnny Pope is one of the greatest story tellers of our time. He is a pastor in Houston and we have been friends for two decades. He shared with me over lunch one time at Cracker Barrel and I will close this chapter with his poignant story. Arturo Toscanini was arguably the greatest musical conductor of his time. He was born in Parma, Italy and was one of the most acclaimed conductors of both the 19th and 20th centuries. He was known for his passion, intensity and his ear to orchestral detail. He was equipped with a photographic memory and was nearly a perfectionist.

Dr. Pope went on to say that we find only three types of ovation. If it is good, folks politely clap. If it is really good an audience will stand and clap (standing ovation) but the rarest of ovations is one that most will never witness in life. If it is really, really good they neither clap nor stand but instead sit in silence. It is an awkward moment because immediately one cannot tell if it bombed or it was, as teens say today, "da bomb!"

Toscanini had a two hundred piece orchestra under his command and crowds came to hear him night after night at venues around the globe. They often closed with "Beethoven's Fifth." Each night they played effortlessly and nearly flawlessly and the audience always approved with a roar almost equivalent to a volcano erupting. The great conductor had witnessed twice in his career the rare, almost impossible third ovation and the orchestra under him or the crowds that came out had never seen it firsthand. On one particular night as they concluded with that classic piece they were rolling and literally on all cylinders. When they finished, like a hammer, they "nailed it."

They always got an enormous ovation and most nights the standing ovation but on this evening it was different. Toscanini recognized it immediately but his orchestra below and the crowd beside him didn't know what had just transpired. An eerie silence filled the auditorium and it was an awkward moment and you could hear a pin drop. Did they bomb or was it something to behold? In the silence it became evident that it was the latter and the crowd sat silently savoring both the surreal and special, knowing something sacred had just transpired.

The third time is the charm but it was the first for everyone else and what took place next infuriated The Maestro. His orchestra, when they finally realized what transpired, began to get arrogant, cocky and a smug pride came across their countenances. Some went as far as to slap each other on the back; two pulled on their suspenders and one had the audacity to stand up and say, "I did it. That piece was all because of me!"

The great Toscanini leaned forward with his face like flint and whispered to his two hundred piece orchestra, "Who is Toscanini?" and then he whispered, "Nobody." Then he looked square into their eyes and added, "and who are you?" and said a little louder that only his team could hear, "Nothing" Then he stood in his tuxedo with his baton pointed towards Heaven and loud enough that the entire crowd could hear, " But Beethoven is everything!"

Now, as he did then, John would say, "Who is John the Baptist? Friends, I am nobody!" He would humbly read the roll call of both the known and forgotten leaders of Christianity and recite: "Who is A.W.Tozer, Charles H. Spurgeon, D.L. Moody, John Wesley, Leonard Ravenhill, Charles Stanley,

Adrian Rogers, E.V. Hill, David Jeremiah, Mother Teresa, Rick Warren, Beth Moore, Sheila Walsh, Tony Evans, Billy Graham (among others) and say with tears, "Something" And with his Bible stretched towards Heaven and with tears streaming down his face the forerunner who ran his race for The One coming soon behind him would shout, " but JESUS is everything!"

Looking back, the wilderness was not just to prepare and promote you but to PROTECT you. If you never had setbacks at the start you would not succeed at the finish. God knows exactly how much adversity it takes before He can put you on His Varsity. He may love us the same but He doesn't use us all the same. The Lord uses not only the blessed but broken and I have witnessed Him use our pain, promotions or both to help carry others out of their pit en route to the Promised Land.

Chapter Four

"The Rolling Stones"

"When others see a Shepherd boy, God may see a king. Even though, your life is filled with ordinary things. In just a moment, God can touch you and everything will change. When others see a Shepherd boy – God may see a king!" Ray Boltz penned the words to that classic contemporary and it rings true today.

On the back lot of Hollywood is pretend but the back lot of history is training grounds for future warriors and winners. David is in the desert and he is young, ambitious and like the other characters thus far in the book, overlooked. He has potential and promise but not on the radar to be picked "most likely to succeed." In fact, if his high school had a year book 3000 BC it would be chiseled "most likely to fail."

He was the runt of the family, the last and considered to be the least. In the dust and dirt we find him slinging stones in his spare time. He crafted a leather strap and picked a couple choice rocks and with sling in hand he began to take aim and fire! The first went wide, the others were wild but his focus never flinched. A fire began to burn within and it no longer concerned him what others on the outside thought. He aimed again and again and his precision got better and the velocity with which he fired got more powerful. He was small in size but he was unbelievably strong in spirit. He has heart and this freshman was on fire! At first glance he was unassuming but be careful because if you underestimated him there was a reason he became undefeated.

David began to set his sights on small prey and wild animals. When he captured and conquered them he got a confidence that comes from honing a

God given gift. He was a boy with a man's skill and he got stronger, wiser and deadly with a sling. He faced lions, tigers and bears (oh my!) and took them all out!! This rejected renegade in private was becoming a future Green Beret in public and there was nothing or no one that intimidated him.

I have learned when you kneel before God you can stand before anyone. Notice how he didn't start out in the Major Leagues but practiced his gift in the Minors. Had he not developed his craft when no one was watching he wouldn't be ready to dominate when everyone was looking! David was rejected by family but respected by God. Sound familiar? Just ask Joseph (Cup of Joe) we shared in Chapter Two. Flavor is a taste made by man but FAVOR is the touch of God. One touch from God changes everything! If that is not your cup of tea than you better switch to Christian cappuccino because that is what Divinity delights and brewed by God.

Several years ago, I preached a sermon "Facing Your Fears with Faith." Perseverance is one of my favorite topics since childhood and God instilled in me a fascination with the subject. Don't talk to me about the individual who inherited a fortune but share with me the story of the person knocked down but who wouldn't stay down! The Rev. Jerry Falwell had a sign in his office that read: "How do you stop that man that won't quit? You can't!" My heart beats to learn of folks who have endured tragedy and turned it into triumph. Their setbacks today became success tomorrow. President John F. Kennedy penned in the Oval Office that the word "crisis" in Chinese is composed of two characters. One represents danger and the other opportunity.

Why is it that when some are faced with an obstacle, half will step up and the others sit down? What makes one flourish and the other fail? Is it in the genes? Is it God? Gatorade, or "guts" – like Gatorade, is it in you? Is it a trait taught or caught by a mentor, coach, teacher or pastor? Why do some succeed and the rest succumb to the pressure to remain in the bleachers as a spectator and not get in the game as a soldier? I've learned stress causes many to break but others to BREAK records.

Much can be attributed to the love, leadership and life lessons from our parents and guardians growing up but it is ironic that you can be born in the same house, hear the wise instruction of the same parent(s) and yet still end up in different destinations or with varying decisions. In 2005, I had the privilege to preach at a large youth event with Casting Crowns and Duffy Robbins. Before the service, it was an honor to eat dinner in the green room and actually play three-on-three basketball with lead singer Mark Hall and Casting Crowns. That will be one evening I will not soon forget.

That evening during the invitation, we had over 100 salvations and Mark (lead singer to Crowns) said, "It is amazing that kids in my youth group will go on a retreat and read the same words on the screen, sit side by side, sing the exact same songs, listen to the same speaker and hang out with the same students but some will embrace the message of God's gospel and others will reject it." Even Christ on the cross learned that some will reject the Gospel and others accept. However, if we don't meet Jesus as the gentle lamb on Earth we will stand before Him as the Lion of Tribe of Judah in Heaven.

The life verse of Tim Heddings, one of my best friends since fourth grade, is 1 Cor. 1:17 "God uses the foolish to confound the wise." God, since the beginning of time, has always used the ordinary to do the extraordinary. Mother Mary was "great" because of God the Father's grace. It was because of His mercy, not her merits, that she has a special place in history and in our hearts. God used Mary's virgin's womb in birth and the virgin tomb of Joseph of Arimathea in death to carry out His plan on the world's stage.

Let's get back to our already scheduled program featuring David in the desert. He seemed neglected by day but was growing more confident at night. We find a fine line between being arrogant and confident. Arrogance depends on you but confidence is totally depending on God. Terror had come to town and fear had gripped the land. Goliath was larger than life and he instilled death and doom to everyone he encountered. It was his way or the highway but up to that point the opposition had no options. It was fall in line existing in life or die trying.

The experts, professionals and elder brothers had grown sick and tired of being sick and tired. The problem was not one of them was willing to take on the giant. Goliath was a mountain of flesh and on the playing field no one had a miniscule of faith. The Bible says: "If we have faith the size of a mustard seed" our obstacles will fumble, mountains crumble and giants tumble before our eyes. The problem was that folks had faith in the boardrooms but not on the gym floor. They dominated in private but failed in public and Goliath arrogantly mocked them as a man among boys. It was appropriate he was arrogant because "pride goes before the fall" and still on the backside of the desert is a boy who is getting ready to topple a massive man and Goliath of a giant.

When the giant walked, the earth shook and men's knees would shake. Their hearts trembled with fear and their palms filled with perspiration. Goliath continued to tout his undefeated record and belittle the band of brothers on the sideline. He challenged with his growl that could be heard clear to Golgotha that he was ready, willing and able to take on anyone and everyone. However, no one moved. He laughed and cocked his head back and took in the sweet victory. This temporal satisfaction gave him all the more reason to taunt and tease his opponents only to demoralize them mentally and stroke his ego personally.

Michael Buffer's distant ancestor with his rich bass voice walked towards the giant and stood in the sandlot. In his Sunday best he pulled a mega phone to his lips and like a bugler getting ready to play "Taps" sounded a clarion call that aroused only Goliath and belted "Let's get ready to Rumble!" Ironically, the opposition heard "let's get ready to FUMBLE" because drop the ball they did. Those clowns from another town died in their tracks, they were the frozen chosen and they lost before the match started. In Rambo II, Stallone said to Murdock: "The greatest weapon is the mind." Henry Ford said: "If you think you can or can't you are right." Jesus said: "As a man thinks so he is." The Bible notes, "A double minded man is unstable in all his ways."

These guys were not wishy-washy because they were stuck in the washer and dryer. In the left corner were hundreds of men dressed as soldiers but who resembled "sissies" and yet some of their sisters had more of a desire to fight. You have heard of the phrase "all dressed up and nowhere to go" that explains this motley crew now in the "yellow" corner. They were afraid, ashamed and scared to advance. When the bell sounded, no one and I mean NO ONE stepped forward. In fact, they took three steps back!

They screamed, Goliath smiled, and out of nowhere stepped forth a man (actually a kid with an adult's fire and a champion's heart). Startled, his colleagues were thinking: "Little David is too small" but at the same time satisfied that somebody, anyone but them was willing to step forward facing this foe despite certain death. Just like on 9/11 when most were running out, the real heroes were running in!

The young shepherd boy grabbed his gear and ran towards the battlefield while everyone else was on the bleachers. Ironically, his fellow soldiers all of a sudden become instant "experts" and coaching him from afar how to fight, yet they have never stepped foot into war. They thought they were seasoned on gorilla (Goliath) warfare and gladly tried to tell him how to face the giant. David declined their advice to take on more equipment to fight the Philistine, informing them that he had not "proven" the gear in preparation for the task at hand. David made up his mind to face Goliath relying on what had worked for him in the past.

David had killed animals and became accurate with his sling, steadily advancing his skills en route to his date with destiny (not his death). Similar to baseball players, one doesn't start out in the Majors but they excelled in the minors only after playing Little League, Parks and Recreation, JV, varsity ball, college ball and maybe A, AA, AAA and if they are fortunate, the call comes for the high honor to play in the Big Leagues!

Despite David's backyard BASIC training, hands down, it was still the greatest mismatch in history. Soldier verses student, old verses young, warrior against a walk on. In a nutshell, a killer of the Armed Forces verses a kid who was a keeper of his father's flock.

David may have looked like Raggedy Ann walking out, but he had Rambo's fire in his eyes and was equipped with a sling and five smooth stones that he picked out. David didn't walk, but rather ran, to the center of the ring. Goliath did what he always did -- he began to taunt him, humiliate him and intimidate this youth from the local YMCA. To this day, callous commentators make fun of Peter for falling out at sea. However, at least he was willing to get out of the boat! I would rather have one Peter out at sea than ten in a boat any day of the week! Dr. Charles Spurgeon was asked how he built the 5,000 member tabernacle and he said, "All I needed were ten men totally surrendered to the will of God."

Absent is Russell Crowe and on the very first set of "Gladiator" was young David. No one gave him a chance and no one uttered a prayer. They were convinced that he couldn't go toe to toe much less the distance with this killing machine. Goliath was a mountain of flesh but David was a mountain of faith! Some on the sidelines thought: "David is so little how can he hurt him?" David, with his childlike faith but warrior spirit was thinking, "Goliath is so big I cannot miss him!" When most saw an obstacle, David saw an amazing opportunity. Today, when others see a crisis do you see Christ? Never stare at the problem at hand but the Answer in your heart (Jesus).

What goes through one's mind during this stand off? Well, let me give you the play by play. Goliath was quoting in advance what Mr. T (Clubber Lang) said in ROCKY III "Dead Meat!" Truth be told, as David was placing his first stone in that sling he was prophetically quoting what Clint Eastwood would say thousands of years later in a Dirty Harry flick, "Do you feel lucky, punk?"

The crowd rallied, Goliath roared and David reared back with his sling and like a heat sinking missile hit its mark exploding and smashing him square in the forehead. For a brief moment, time stood still. The crowd hushed, David rushed and Goliath didn't have time to blush because his face had turned from danger red to ashen white. His knees buckled and the giant fell to the ground with a loud BOOM never to get up. The Earth shook and the Heavens shouted, "Glory to the God in the Highest!" For a brief moment we have peace on Earth and goodwill toward men. When others see a shepherd boy, God truly saw a king" and David knew first hand "the bigger they are the harder they fall." David's future son could clearly say: "Papa was a rolling stone!"

It always was intriguing to me that David selected five smooth stones. For starters, most wouldn't think he could fire the first one off. Secondly, if he did and missed, it would be over before he could reload the second stone. I am convinced that he didn't pack five in his arsenal in case he missed but because we learn a Biblical fact that Goliath had four other brothers and David was willing to take them all out – one at a time! Never judge a book by its cover because Goliath was once undefeated but it's the lad who is now undisputed.

David won the battle years before in his mind while tending his Daddy's sheep. That day, he didn't come to merely dance but to dominate! He didn't come to fight but to finish the work God called him to do. He didn't have a victim mindset but knew intimately that he was already the victor in Almighty God.

Goliath was arrogant and David was totally dependent on God. Goliath died in the flesh but David lived another day by faith. David was not content with mediocrity ministry but he was destined to be a soldier in the Lord's Army not some bum sitting on the sidelines. He knew with God above, around, beside and best of all, in him, he couldn't lose! The hardest part was practicing in private and showing up publicly on game day. Sometimes the hardest part of success is showing up.

While a student in high school nearly twenty-five years ago, it was my honor to prepare and occasionally teach Sunday school at First Baptist Church of Waldorf, MD. I used to beat myself up because just as David had only five smooth stones, early on in my ministry I felt like I only had five smooth sermons. It was tempting to quit and throw in the towel. Satan would tease me and tell me repeatedly to forsake the call on my life because I didn't have more messages. However, God reminded me that the Word doesn't return void and you can only sling one sermon at a time. Even today, those sermons still slay giants every single time when slung with the Spirit of God behind them.

David knew absent God he couldn't win, but with God he couldn't fail. With eyes of faith, David saw past the natural and got a glimpse of the supernatural. God is still on the lookout for folks to be giant killers, those who dare to be a Daniel against a den of lions, a David against all odds in this game called life. Folks like Shadrach, Meshach and Abednego who would rather burn for Jesus than be "watered down" without Him!

Courage is moving forward in faith even when it doesn't feel comfortable or convenient. Christianity is not emotion but devotion. The day Goliath dropped dead, David ran on top of him and with the giant's own sword, cut off his head. Ironically, Goliath had already lost his mind when he thought he could live life without the Lord. Both John the Baptist and Goliath lost their heads. John was killed for honoring God. Goliath lost his for dishonoring God and trying to touch His anointed.

David, without question, was carrying greatness. However, the value was not in his hand (sling or stone) but in his head and heart where his Savior permeated his thinking. David was carrying greatness but greatness was both carrying and compelling him forward. He had a date with destiny and on that day only one was going to be dead and David did more than die trying. He knew death had no sting when equipped with Holy Spirit stones and sling.

Sylvester Stallone often signs his autograph, "Keep Punching" and may we all keep swinging for Jesus. David was once at a rock and a hard place but once he trusted God and used his gift for His glory, then Goliath found on his forehead that rock and hit him hard. Stay confident in Christ and be mindful that pride comes before the fall.

CHAPTER FIVE

"WILD IN WINSTON-SALEM"

It was 1993, and my pastor told me that I absolutely needed to attend a pastor's conference in Winston-Salem, North Carolina. The catch is the trip was 48 hours away and would last five days and four nights. It was an 800 mile round trip trek and I had no place to stay and the real kicker was I had $65.00!

The clock was ticking and it was obvious God gave me more faith than finances and I don't know what you would have done, but my buddy Tim and I left Maryland in my 1983 Datsun 280ZX and with the lyrics of James Taylor dancing in my head I heard, "In My Mind I'm Going to Carolina!" Appropriately, my vanity tags on my car were "Z U L8R" and God said "go" and we were gone!

I recall hearing when Michael Jordan was cut from the varsity basketball team at Laney High in Wilmington, NC he ran to his room and cried for three days. When he finally came out he approached the coach and asked to be the ball boy. His coach said, "Mike, you are not that bad and you don't have to degrade yourself to do that. Perhaps next year you will make the team." Mike heard enough and said, "Coach, I just have to be around it."

With a Z and a prayer we rolled south and I didn't have a place to stay but just knew that I had to be around the preaching and atmosphere. If it meant sleeping in my car for the first time in my life I was willing to be homeless just to soak up the sermons and sit in the anointing of some of the greatest preachers of that generation. Keep in mind, $65.00 had to cover gas to travel 800 miles; twelve meals (three a day times four); and no hotel accommodations. Mathematically, it was impossible.

God indeed had fed five thousand one night and four thousand another and perhaps He would have mercy on us two poor souls and feed us. However, I also recall reading in the Bible that Jesus was so immersed in His Father's business that His disciples tried to get Him to eat and He said, "I have food that you know not of." My prayer was that perhaps we would be so HUNGRY for God that food would be an afterthought. Either way, like Smokey and the Bandit, we had a long way to go and a short time to get there! We were not only driving fast but most likely we would be fasting all the way down Interstate 85 South for the next week.

Sometimes folks see your public platform today but don't take inventory of your private pain or the price it took along the way yesterday. They see the stage but not your scars en route to climbing the steps of the platform. Favor comes after faith even in the dictionary and I am certain of show me your faith and I will show you your future. Others may be more gifted, talented and connected but if you have more faith you will run circles around them ALL day long. This is not arrogant but an accurate assessment, because without faith it is IMPOSSIBLE to please God. You cannot buy success or manufacture obedience. The road to success is paved with many toll booths but the key are you willing to trust God because He has already paid the price? Most of us have more head knowledge than heart application anyway. Where the rubber meets the road is when we graduate from the couch and buckle up and roll on for God's glory.

That seven hour trip south was one of the best days of my life. We were young, hungry, broke but obedient. Looking back, that is not a bad place to be. The problem is when we rely more on our savings than Savior and more on our checking account than on Christ Almighty. Finances are good but faith in God will win all day long!

The conference was to be held at Gospel Light Baptist Church in Walkertown, NC, just outside of Winston-Salem. As long as I live, I will never forget what transpired next. We were just ten miles from the conference with not much time to spare and were still an hour out before it began. Keep in mind we had $65 to last five days and four nights!

We got off an exit in Winston-Salem and what transpired next was WILD! It was almost as if we were in the Bermuda Triangle and my car was sucked into an abyss. Not into a hole but into a hotel! It was the five-star Grand Marquee Hotel. What are two 21 year olds from Maryland with next to no money doing driving into the parking lot of this grand hotel? It made even less sense when we proceeded to waltz into the lobby (because we had neither dollars nor cents)! The lobby was filled to the gills with men in nice business suits and I recall it being one of the first ever glass elevators I had ever seen. For a split second, I thought we were in California and we were now the Beverly Hillbillies!

With Tim in tow, I approached the front desk and what transpired next made even less sense. At this point, I can only explain it was out of character and I felt as if I was a pawn on God's chess board because at this point it was not me and had to be ALL Him. Fresh from driving seven hours and 400 miles I inquired how much for a room? Hello!! Don't forget I am in a five star hotel, minutes from the start of the conference with next to NO money and I am asking how much for a room? Plus, time is ticking and why are we even there?

The man stared me up and down and said sarcastically, "We are SOLD OUT!" We have been for two months because of a preachers' conference in town. The way he said it with a snarl made me think he wasn't a brother in the Lord. Ironically, I am trying to save money but now concerned if his soul is saved. The capacity crowd explained that some of the nicely dressed men in suits may have been clergy. He proceeded to stare me up and down and if looks could kill he murdered me in the lobby of that hotel.

He said, "Where are you from?" I replied: "Sir, I am from Maryland." He asked why I was in town and I said "Actually, to attend the preachers' conference." His mouth dropped because I probably was not only the youngest to attend but probably drove the furthest to get there. He then dug deeper with disgust and said, "Let me get this straight, you drove seven hours and four hundred miles for a preachers' conference and you are ill prepared and you don't have a place to stay?" Now thinking I let God down because I had the faith to leave Maryland but didn't quite get the entire week planned out while in Carolina, replied almost embarrassingly, "yes sir." He was stunned and I felt undone. I knew it was going to be a long week and I had signed up for this and humbly walked away towards the door and told Tim, "let's get going" and we were heading back towards the parking lot for my "Z".

En route to the rotating glass door to leave the hotel lobby, the desk clerk called me back. Honestly, I didn't feel like being verbally assaulted again nor having God look worse with my poor Christian witness for "not being prepared." Reluctantly, I retraced my steps and what he said was like music to my ears. "Mr. Shelton, I don't know why I am telling you this because I have never done it before and most likely will never do it again."

He had my undivided attention. He said, "Technically we are sold out and technically we are not." I said: "Sir, you sound like a lawyer, please share what technically means?" He said: "As a perk to our employees we always keep one room available in case they have out of town family to accommodate them at our hotel. Even though we may advertise "sold out" we usually have a spare room." I knew curiosity killed cats but I was willing to hear the rest of what he had to say regardless if he made fun of my faith or not.

The man stared at me up and down one more time but this time it was not in disgust or disdain but almost disbelief and respect on his part. His face was no longer contorted but compassionate and he said something that echoes in my ears today, exactly two decades later. He said, "Young man, you are on a mission from God, aren't you?" All I could think of was John Belushi and Dan Aykroyd as the Blues Brothers came to mind and dancing in my head was "I'm a Soul Man!" No joke, this Baptist almost began to break dance right on the marble floor of the Grand Marquee adorned with glass elevators and all!

As if eternity had passed, but not missing a millisecond, I said, "Sir, I guess I am." This atheist was now a believer if not in God but in us glorified goofballs from Maryland and he said these words, "Mr. Shelton, here is what I am going to do. I am going to give you the room for $49." My first reaction was PRAISE THE LORD because that means only three nights in the "Z." My A.D.D. kicked in thinking I don't know what we are going to do for food but at least we get one good night's rest while in North Carolina! Keep in mind, we never talked money and he didn't know how much or little we had. When I inquired was that $49 per night he said "no, it's $49 for the duration of your stay." At this point, I almost fell back. I am not Pentecostal but almost fell out in the Spirit right then and there!

Trying to be gracious but not overly surprised we thanked him and tried to contain ourselves in the lobby because after all we were two kids in a hotel that was way out of our league. We got in the glass elevator and still had to maintain our composure because we had to represent Christ and truth be told they Windex the windows of the elevator on the hour and just knew his and every other pair of eyes were still staring at us. Previously, he stared me down and now had the suspicion they were staring at us going up. Before I had thought of James Taylor with "Carolina on my Mind" and just recently had the Blues Brother's theme song, "I am a Soul Man". Now heading towards Heaven, all I could think of was the theme song of George Jefferson's TV show "Moving on UP!"

We turned left off the elevator, still in awe of what God just did for us and put the key in the door. Once we walked in, turned around and closed the door, we began to high five each other and almost fell on the floor laughing as if we just won the lottery! I looked on the back of the hotel door and it had a room rate affixed on the back and it read $249 PER NIGHT! That is $1,000 worth of a room (four nights) for $49! God knocked our socks off and like two kids in a candy store we jumped on the bed and celebrated again what God did in our midst.

It dawned on us that we had just ten minutes to drive ten miles to the conference and in the midst of the celebration we almost forget why we came in the first place -- to attend the conference! We got cleaned up, back on the glass elevator and heading down to the lobby and we were on cloud nine. Time was ticking, people were watching and we were racing to the car to get our praise on.

Now the entire lobby had cleared out and en route to the car I noticed one elderly man leaning against a chair all alone. He was distinguished looking, appeared to be in his eighties and had snow white hair. He was wearing a sharp, navy blue double breasted suit and a dark tie. Honestly, he looked like a United States Senator, but in my spirit I thought he may not be a Christian. One can have wealth but if your worth isn't in Jesus then you are broke.

If I ever heard the voice of God, I felt like the Holy Spirit impressed in me to invite the man to church. The worse he could say was "no." We are two kids, three states away from our homes, inviting a first time visitor to a church we don't belong to, or have never been to! I tell folks today all across America, "I don't evangelize because I am an evangelist but because I am a committed Christian." Tim was already out the door and telling me to "come on" and I just had to ask the elderly gentleman if he would be our guest. He looked at me and with the softest eyes and sweetest smile said, "Indeed, I would!" My first reaction in my mind was "Praise God this brother is going to get saved!"

With God above, Tim out front and my new senior citizen behind, we are now headed to the "Z." When you are young and single most men pride themselves on their car. Yes, my car was clean and I had washed and waxed it, and had the wheels shining in the sun with enough Armor All to make the tires glean darker than the Carolina tar pavement.

Tim, all 6"4, selflessly climbed in the back of my 2+2 that could accommodate a bag of groceries at best and our new friend gingerly sat shotgun. With no time to spare, we were racing to the preachers' conference. While driving I kept praying silently that this gentleman would trust Christ as Savior but the more I drove I had this strange suspicion that he might be someone special. Perhaps important and he had this grace and aura about him but I couldn't figure it out. I just know God said invite him and I did!

The church holds 2,500 with the balcony and when we pulled up in the parking lot almost every spot was already taken. I noticed a few stragglers en route to the church but something peculiar happened when they saw my car. Almost everyone stopped and circled my car like a shark around its bleeding prey in the water. What was even more interesting is they didn't come to the driver side of the car but to the passenger. My initial thought was "my car is clean but NOT that clean!"

Friends, I am so slow it takes me two hours to watch "60 Minutes!" The crowd came to his side of the car and when the door opened they shoved their Bibles in his lap begging him to sign them. At this time, I started thinking this brother might already be a Christian! Confused but not trying to look any dumber I felt like a two man Secret Service detail assigned to protect the president but honestly we didn't know the name of the principal we were assisting! I definitely didn't want to blow our cover and look clueless because we had a reputation to uphold!

This saintly senior was now in his element and he gracefully glided across the parking lot and headed straight to the church. When the crowd inside the church saw him approaching the glass doors they immediately opened them with joy. The conference had already started and I bet there were hundreds in the overflow of that church hallway. However, when they saw us with him it was just like the parting of the Red Sea. At this juncture I finally figured out who we had with us. My initial thought it was either Charlton Heston or Moses because I have never seen this happen but I knew this brother was special. We weren't sure what it was but he certainly carried greatness! I didn't know his name but knew that he was different.

My friends back home call me "special" too. They say "birds of a feather flock together." Someone opened the door to the sanctuary and I was just thinking if there are three hundred out here then there must certainly be no room inside! Sure enough when we walked in the first thing I noticed that it was standing room only. People were hanging over the balcony, the place was packed and the choir was just finishing singing. An usher escorted us down the right side of the sanctuary and he does the unthinkable. He takes us towards the front but from my advantage point there were no seats whatsoever anywhere in that cavernous auditorium.

Just an hour before it seemed like all eyes were on us in the hotel but now literally 5,000 eye balls were glued to us. Even if Ray Charles were in the house that blind brother would be staring at us. While we were following the usher and our new friend (aka Moses) and darn if they didn't put us in the FRONT ROW! I felt like Bob Uecker and God taught me years ago, "Those who travel the furthest go the farthest." God has a way to grant gracious nuggets from Heaven to encourage us occasionally in our walk on Earth.

Dr. Curtis Hutson was the moderator of the conference and in front of two thousand plus souls he said these words, "Tonight, our keynote speaker has been in the ministry for 65 years, he has baptized 63,000 souls and is an international evangelist and president emeritus of Tennessee Temple University in Chattanooga, TN. Would you please give a warm Walkertown welcome to Dr. Lee Roberson!" The church came unglued, the crowd gave a standing ovation and the man sitting next to me whom I drove in my car, got up and walked towards the platform! At this juncture my buddy, Tim and I literally fell on the floor!

What Dr. Roberson did next spoke volumes and as he looked to the capacity crowd turned his eyes off thousands and gazed towards Tim and me as individuals. He said, "I want to thank the two young men from Maryland who drove me here tonight because if it were not for them I wouldn't be here this evening." Tim stood up and faced the crowd and said, "He's talking about us! He's talking about us!!" About this time, I had to grab Tim and silence him thinking the guest speaker was going to preach on humility.

Looking back what is comical but was all Christ is the fact that the man who was supposed to pick up the Dr. Billy Graham of that denomination never made it to the hotel that night. When God asked me to invite him, I was thinking it was to see him be saved but God had other plans. Immediately following the service, despite a crowd circling him like a lunch line at Chick-fil-A, Dr. Roberson gravitated towards us and asked if we would chaperone him the rest of the week. Mom always said: "Dance with the one who took you to the prom." Yes, I am slow but didn't have to pray about that and said, "I will take you wherever you want to go."

God blessed us again because by driving Dr. Roberson we not only got to spend precious time with him but also got to dine with him two meals per day. All the other countless clergy in between workshop sessions would go out to eat at local restaurants but we were hand selected to accompany Dr. Roberson to dine with the other four speakers of that pastors' conference. The group included Dr. Jack Hyles, Dr. Curtis Hutson, Dr. Clyde Box, Dr. R.B. Oulette and of course, our new best friend, Dr. Lee Roberson! Today, that would have been equivalent to Dr. Charles Stanley, Dr. Adrian Rogers, Dr. Billy Graham, Dr. Johnny Hunt and Dr. Jack Graham at the table of the inner circle. It may have been broad daylight but they were the "knights of the round table" to me. They were Lancelot and I was Lancelot Link the secret chimp! To say it was "tall cotton" was an understatement!

Honestly, I am not sure if God impressed on him to invite us because he felt sorry for us, to reward us, or if it was so plain obvious that we were running low on financial fumes? All I know is that we honored God and God honored us! Our faith was at an all time high and as if that wasn't enough, God then topped off our tank. We not only got to eat two of the three meals a day free, but we had the honor of dining at the table with the big boys, who were our heroes of the faith! Show me your faith and I will show you your future. God's favor sometimes is released after our faith.

When we finally made it back to the hotel that night it was already late. But when you are ON FIRE for God and filled with the Holy Ghost you cannot sleep nor contain it and you lose track of time. It was well past midnight but we just had to call our pastor who had encouraged us to attend.

He answered the phone in his soft voice not to wake his wife and we were screaming in the phone, "Pastor, you are not going to believe what God did down here. He gave us a hotel room plus we're eating for free and having the time of our lives! Promise us now you will get in the car and drive seven hours tomorrow to meet us at this conference." Without missing a beat and still half asleep he replied: "Guys, you are in front of nearly three thousand people and even if I come how will I ever find you?" I screamed with a laugh, "It's easy! Look for the heavy weights and we are driving them to the service and most likely standing right next to them!"

To pastor's credit, he also made the 400 mile trek and for the next three days joined us and we had a time! You cannot out give God! Almost twenty years to the date, I was invited back to preach just outside of Winston-Salem. A local Baptist church flew me in to preach their revival and it dawned on me that since that conference I have been blessed to preach from coast to coast of North Carolina but this was the first time I had returned to Winston-Salem since that faith-filled trip. The first time I was driving the evangelist but today they were flying me in as the evangelist!

It was my high honor to reunite one more time with Dr. Lee Roberson before his passing. Initially I thought I was driving him but it was really God and Dr. Roberson who were driving me. Often I sit back and ponder how many people with funds or not would have had the faith to be obedient to God and take the 800 mile round-trip with only $65.00? All I knew was just like

Michael Jordan with a basketball, I on a smaller scale, just had to be around the atmosphere and anointing even if it meant sleeping in the car, no food or not certain to have enough gas to get home. We walk by faith and not by sight and we may have hitchhiked home but it would have been better to trust God by faith than to trust man's finances. Humans get stuck in the impossible but with God all things are possible!

Without question, God gives second and third chances and allows us to re-take tests but I often shudder to think what if I had stayed on the couch, didn't trust God or have the faith to get up, walk out and drive down to North Carolina. Who in their wildest dreams would have guessed that God would have done all that for two boys who were too dumb to doubt but smart enough to know that Jesus can be trusted.

Today, I am no Dr. Lee Roberson, but I am an evangelist crisscrossing America and around the Globe. This year alone, I have been in all 48 of the continental United States and preached on world-wide television on numerous outlets from TBN, Daystar, Fox News among others. I will be the first to tell you it is all God and by His grace. It has been said, "Who you hang with is what you become" and I pray that God is pleased and my parents and Dr. Roberson are proud.

If I didn't make it to North Carolina I'm not sure if I would have been everywhere else. The trip to Winston-Salem lit a fire in my heart and provided wind to my sails that truly with God all things are possible. When He guides – He provides and when we are in His will it is on His bill. It is our responsibility to be obedient and it's His job to provide. God blessed us with an amazing hotel, free food and even a seat at the table with our heroes, fellowship that comes from only clean living and honoring Christ, and memories that would last a million miles!

The moment I met Dr. Lee Roberson I knew he was unique and special. Regardless if he were saved or lost, I knew he had class and clout. When we drove him to the event I just knew I had someone special in my car, and I am not the sharpest tool in the shed but I knew then what I know now -- we were blessed to carry greatness! Thank you, Jesus!

CHAPTER SIX

"LEMON – AIDE"

At one time I felt like if they had a sequel to Tom Hank's iconic role "Forest Gump" I could probably play him but the fact is I would do better to be in the prequel. Sometimes I can't help but smile and laugh out loud because my friends think I was "Forest Gump" even before there was "Forest Gump."

Regardless, whether I was spending the weekend as a teen in Beverly Hills, California with the biggest action star in Hollywood history, Sly Stallone or running into and working for multiple U.S. Presidents, driving Grammy Winners and future governors in my car, working as a personal assistant to Members of Congress or spending the night as friends with former World Wrestling Champions it has been a wild ride and all God.

My first encounter with the legendary and world famous Harlem Globetrotters came when I was in elementary school and I used to watch them periodically on Wide World of Sports on Saturday on television. Their iconic red, white and blue jerseys were priceless and I still think their shorts resembled Apollo Creed's boxing trunks in the first ROCKY movie. My fourth grade friend Joe asked a couple of us one day at recess in elementary school if we wanted to buy replica uniforms of my favorite basketball team.

The answer was a resounding "YES" but I didn't know how much they would cost. Joe was my classmate but already quite the promoter and he said he could get them in 1982 for about ten bucks. For a kid in elementary school that was possible and I began to volunteer to take out the trash, cut the yard, rake leaves, wash the car, collect soda cans and even looked under the sofa for any loose change. After saving up my money I gave it to Joe with hopes of getting my very own basketball uniform to match my heroes!

Most kids run away from the school bus but I actually raced to it just to ask Joe daily "Did they come in?" Day after day, week after week and month after month I got excuse after excuse. Joe is a great guy and my best friend at that time but he was good at promoting but just a little off on the delivery. He resembled a politician. All promises but no solution. Thank God he wasn't a future Domino's Pizza delivery man or UPS driver because his personality was second to none but his follow through was less than first rate. Frankly, you may never get your pizza or product.

Well, fourth grade came and went but I will still holding out hope for my Globetrotter uniform to come in. The next year I graduated from fifth grade with a paper diploma but no red, white and blue Globetrotter jersey. Joe moved out of town and I kind of felt rejected. No friend and no follow through. Did it get lost in the mail, did it even exist or was it too good to be true? I never held it against Joe but that jersey would have been cool and I still believe that a friendship is more valuable than fame, fortune or the famed replica uniform.

Two years later, basketball began to be a big part of my life. I was playing on various basketball teams and for a white guy near the Nation's Capital it was a help to meet friends if you could play ball. Plus, it taught great teamwork. One of my best friends was Patrick Cottman and he was black and they tell me I am white.

Together, we were "Ebony & Ivory" in the halls of school and hardwood on the court. At the time, he was leading scorer for our team and I was a close second. We often spent the night over each other's house that seventh and eighth grade year. His mother was a divorcee and she did a fine job raising Pat on her own. He was well liked, a great ball player and super guy.

He called me one day and said: "Frank, my mother won a radio contest today!" It was a respected African American radio station and she got three complimentary tickets to see the legendary Harlem Globetrotters. It got better! He then said: "The tickets note there will be a free basketball clinic two hours before the game and you can interact and meet the team and play on

the floor of the NBA Washington Bullets at the now defunct Capital Centre."
He then proceeded to ask: "Do you want to come?" Do I want to come?! In
the words of Balboa himself: "Absolutely!"

The next weekend couldn't get here soon enough and when you are a kid
you tend to have a one track mind. The year is 1985 and I just turned 13
and we are en route to the Capital Centre. It was an NBA court and seated
18,000. Ironically, I saw Elvis Presley perform one of his last concerts in the
same arena just two months before he died in 1977. Now I was playing on
the big stage with the big boys! It reminded me later of Dr. Lee Roberson and
his Bible. Go God!

Only the Creator of the Universe could write this script. We arrived and
it was bone cold outside but we were warm with hoop dreams. They ushered
us towards the front just a couple rows from the floor and we were beyond
a kid in the candy store. When you are barely a teen and sitting this close to
greatness it's almost surreal. We heard basketballs bouncing from the other
side of that massive arena and it was almost empty except a couple janitors
cleaning the venue before the doors opened to the general public.

We not only heard balls bouncing but shoes squeaking and that trademark
laugh. My head couldn't turn quick enough and it was none other than the
Harlem Globetrotters coming out playing tricks, high five those of us in the
stands and adorning smiles wider than the state of Maryland. Better yet,
they were coming single file over towards us! A representative from the radio
station gave a brief introduction and there in the flesh was one of my heroes
and the greatest dribblers the game ever produced, Curly Neale.

A whistle blew and it was one of the referees who would cover the game
later that day and then said music to our ears, "Come on to the floor!" They
didn't have to call me twice and Patrick and I jumped on the floor. I will never
forget the feeling of walking on that professional basketball court. It was
almost as if I felt like anything could be possible from that moment on. Why
did these "God moments" keep happening to me? The Bible does tell us, "If
we delight in the Lord He gives us the desires of our heart." I was not using
God to get stuff but He sure was gracious to me!

At this juncture the thought of Joe from elementary school failing to deliver my Globetrotter jersey was out the window. Especially, when you are now on the floor shooting hoops with them! The reason our rear view window is smaller than the car windshield is because where we are going is more important than where we have been. If we keep looking in reverse we will fail to appreciate the present and crash in the future.

That afternoon we played a mini game and they taught us various ball handing and defensive exercises and I recall the first time I shot a free throw on that massive, professional court. The basketball literally disappeared into the night and out of nowhere came back down and swished through the net! I had never played in such a massive arena before and my eyes were not acclimated to the vastness of that arena.

God enabled us to make memories that will last a lifetime and we went back into the stands and watched our heroes dominate the Washington Generals immediately after our clinic. It was almost comical that they tried to teach us defense because I don't recall either team playing much defense that game but it was definitely more fun than fundamentals and they truly are some of the best in the world.

I thanked Patrick's mom profusely and life was good. Upon graduating from middle school, I went on to play three years for Thomas Stone High basketball team and they lost the State Championship my sophomore year. Upon graduation, I contemplated playing a season or two at the community college before transferring to a Christian university in North Carolina but elected to coach youth basketball for Parks and Recreation. We had a great time and I began to speak and minister on the side locally while at home.

As if it were yesterday, I recall watching a television program and the guest speaker was my hero, Meadowlark Lemon. He is the Clown Prince of Basketball and in millions of fans' estimation "THE Harlem Globetrotter." He has played in 18,000 consecutive games and now inducted 2003, in the Basketball Hall of Fame. He was on a Gaither Homecoming Special and sharing his testimony of his faith in Christ. When I heard that he was born-again I jumped off the couch with tears of JOY to hear that one of my heroes was now a kid of The King! Plus, it thrilled my heart that he was now a minister of the Gospel!

I began to follow him again from afar with both basketball and his Bible and found his website. The worse someone can say is "no" and delay now doesn't mean denial later. We found his information and inquired to see if we could ever bring him to my hometown. The timing didn't work out the first time but out of the blue I got a call from his assistant in Arizona and she shared that Meadowlark was coming to Washington, D.C. and could I help get him in a local church?

God opened the door and the day arrived that I would be face to face with my childhood hero. Meadowlark accepted our invite and he came to preach at a local Baptist Church in Maryland. We reunited privately in the pastor's study and we filmed a video together and when we uploaded it on YouTube we got tons of traction and feedback! He did a super job that day, signed countless basketballs and brought the House down with his joy and message on Jesus.

Without a doubt, he is a crowd favorite wherever he goes and he is one of the few people known around the world by his first name! They say "birds of feather flock together" and He is Meadowlark and he calls me "parakeet." I am no eagle but praise God that His eye is on the sparrow!

After signing every item, he had to leave for another engagement that night in Washington and he was whisked away. What a treat it was to catch up with him after all these years! We exchanged pleasantries and phone numbers and occasionally stayed in touch. He is not only the consummate showman but also a class act and the king of correspondence. I learned that the greats are gracious.

Several months later, I was checking emails around midnight and what I received next I had to read and re-read two or three times. It was from his office and his assistant was telling me his new book was to be released in a couple months and Meadowlark was inquiring if I would write a testimonial and submit one of the forewords to his book entitled, Trust Your Next Shot. What an honor!

That night I cranked it out and wanted to make sure it was just right and I couldn't believe that a living legend would want something from little me. The book became a great success because Meadowlark had lived a life of class and contribution. He got tons of great press from his book and David Letterman had him fly back to New York City to promote it on his show. Letterman couldn't have been more pleased to be in Meadowlark's presence but then again it was that way with almost everyone.

President Obama, when he was still a sitting United States Senator, submitted his foreword to the book along with NBA great Michael Jordan and comedian Bill Cosby and now also the glorified goofball from Southern Maryland, yours truly! What an honor it was to be linked with greatness.

About a year later, I got a call from his assistant again and she shared that Meadowlark would be back in Washington D.C. and could I assist getting him into some schools or churches? When your heroes call you cannot but want to help. I have always said it is one of life's greatest pleasures to go from a fan to friend but this friend is still one of his biggest fans! I worked my rolodex and began to try to open doors for Meadowlark and we got him in three more churches. At each event, he asked me to introduce him before he spoke. I realized what you do for others God may do for you.

My intent was to promote him but God and Meadowlark promoted me in the process. We will never see a harvest in our business, endeavors or ministry until we sacrificially sow into another's first. We spent more time together and I was his chaperone, chauffer and closest assistant while near Capitol Hill.

He began to mail me boxes of those iconic red, white and blue basketballs in advance and I would have the fun task of blowing them all up before his arrival. They would be neatly displayed at the product table and folks would pay for him to sign the basketballs. Our friendship grew closer and we would grab meals together and it dawned on me that I am now sitting across the table and sharing the stage while introducing my childhood hero!

We shared many laughs together and after one visit to my hometown it was my time to retrieve him early the next morning at the hotel and transport him to Ronald Reagan National Airport in Washington, D.C. He was going to fly to New York and was a scheduled guest that night on Sean Hannity's show in Fox News studios.

One doesn't have to be a Rhodes Scholar or the sharpest tool in the shed to realize that Meadowlark is special. Not only special but super special and call me crazy but I had this feeling that it was my honor to carry greatness. It was as if he was a package on loan from God and He and his wife were subliminally telling me to "handle with care." Meadowlark is joy personified and everyone recognizes him immediately.

It was a cold winter morning in Washington, D.C. and truthfully, I was slightly nervous. For awhile I was my Congressman's fulltime driver and we had been around quite a few folks from Cabinet Members, White House staff to nationally known public officials but something was slightly different each time being around Meadowlark. That morning I pulled up to the curb and I wanted to give him the valet, first class curb service. Quickly, I jumped out of Ruth's black Lincoln SUV and went to go around the other side of the vehicle to grab his luggage and hold the door for him. After all we all have greatness in us and I was trying to honor him.

The car was running and it was cold outside but I wanted to try to close the door without shutting it. Somehow in the transition to help him my door closed and Meadowlark despite being accustomed to being in the presence of Presidents and royal Queens didn't need the fanfare or demand the service. My honest desire was to honor and serve and went to open his door but he beat me to it and already standing outside on the curb of Ronald Reagan National Airport (a friend of his from the past) and he shut his door while reaching to retrieve his own luggage from the passenger rear door. My desire was to open both his door and grab his luggage for him to catch his flight. After all, I knew I was "carrying greatness."

The problem was for some reason the automatic locks were on and with the engine running and my keys in the ignition. I about died right there in front of U.S. Airways curb-side check in. What were the odds? His leather coat was in the back seat and I still have none of his luggage in hand because it was locked in the car! I was trying to help but now only hurt my hero's schedule.

We both looked at each other and I said a "silent prayer" and I felt like the world's biggest loser. All I wanted to do was serve and then this happened. Time was ticking and Meadowlark was the consummate gentleman. The catch is we are not supposed to leave the car parked next to a terminal these days after 9/11. People get nervous quick especially the airport security and it didn't help to have the car running while locked. That wasn't super smart on my part but he was patient and personable and then he flashed me that trademark smile and I knew it was going to be all right.

His plane was boarding within the hour and I didn't have time to call Ruth or a locksmith and it was tempting to break the window just to assist him. However, God reminded me that I had stored the security combination to the door locks on my cell. The car was still new to us and hadn't memorized or even needed to use the codes. Sure enough, cooler heads prevailed and God answered this clown's prayer and the Clown Prince of Basketball got his gear, gave me a big hug and then said: "I love you brother!"

Sadly, racial tension still exists around the world but I wish the cameras could see the friends that I have been blessed to meet and connect with. God has been too good to this goofball. As Meadowlark gracefully entered the terminal it was still fun on the curb to see how all the baggage claim personnel to professional businessmen in suits and pilots stopped almost in awe to see him walk down the hall and darn if he didn't smile or wave to every single one of them. In a world of cubic zirconias he's the genuine article.

While he was in the Big Apple we were watching for him later that evening on Fox News. It is amazing how many people one can connect with in just a single business day and I am convinced he hasn't wasted too many opportunities in life to bless others. We kept in touch on occasion and then I got a call from his wife informing me that he was coming back to D.C. and I assumed he wanted me to chaperone him from event to event. I certainly did not mind and it was an honor to be around him much less serve but then she floored me. She said: "Frank, he doesn't need you to drive but he is in town for two days doing several events and a limousine has been provided but he wants to know if you want to accompany him while in town?"

Let's just say I didn't have to pray too hard for that request! The next thing I knew I am meeting him at his fancy hotel in Arlington, Virginia and who was waiting in the lobby but the ever classy former Globetrotter icon. He gave me a big hug and we picked up where we left off without missing a beat. We jumped in the awaiting black limousine and once again it seemed like all eyes were on us. Truthfully, my goal was never to be seen but that others could hear what God can do! People need the Lord because He is not a way to Heaven but the Only Way.

The limo pulled out and we headed towards Washington. Thinking back, I was reminded that before I was driving Meadowlark, but really, like Dr. Lee Roberson, he was driving us. Even better, on that day Meadowlark and I have a personal chauffer driving us both! I have always said, "When you bless others they often return to take you along for a future ride." Literally!

Our first stop was my favorite building in the whole world, the United States Capitol Building. The same place that I was literally almost born to work in and had been in the hallways of those hallowed halls since my memory will allow me to recall. My mom shared that while she worked at the U.S. Capitol Historical Society that she thought she was going to go into labor with me in corridors of Congress. Most people come from all over the nation to visit or win a seat but very few were "born to work there."

To this day, I still have a United States Senate identification photo that their Human Resources staff made for me when I visited my Dad at work when I was a kid. Plus, having worked there over four different decades, it is truly home away from home.

My Dad served on the United States Capitol Police for 26 years, retiring as Deputy Chief of the department in 1995. During his career, he protected U.S. Presidents, Members of Congress, staff members and tourists while serving on a number of special assignments. As Chairman of the U.S. Capitol Police Inaugural Task Force, he was responsible for the security at the swearing in ceremony for President Clinton's Inauguration on January 20, 1993. As Chairman of the x-ray inspection evaluation process, he assessed the security threats and managed the procurement and installation of the x-ray machines around the Capitol complex and Congressional Office Buildings. As Chairman of the Capitol Police Headquarters Building Design Committee, he was instrumental in the design, construction of and transition to the new police headquarters building. It was a multi-million dollar project and fellow law enforcement called the new station "Shelton Sheraton." Not bad for a police officer! Go Dad!!

As we stared at the United States Capitol and talked in the limo we were waiting for the event to start on the lawn of the West Front. Once it was time to start an event organizer approached the car and gave us the cue to go out and once again Meadowlark dazzled the crowd and when it was done we began to walk together towards the National Mall. Once again, it was surreal that I would be walking with my hero and friend and I felt like Forrest Gump. Perhaps he (Forrest) felt like me?

En route to the Lincoln Memorial we made a brief detour to the new Martin Luther King Memorial. We took a picture of the two of us at the base of the statue and I felt so unworthy to be in that shot because both he and Dr. King were GIANTS. They were known around the world, both fought for racial freedom as goodwill ambassadors and it was grace that I was even in their zip code. I have learned two things: The greats are gracious and when you carry greatness and greatness carries you there are no limits to where God will take you."

We both began to get a tad tired and the limo came up behind us while fans were taking their pictures of Meadowlark entering the car and we dashed off to look for brunch. He asked for my lunch recommendation and we stopped at one of my favorites, the Old Ebbitt Grill, which is next door to the White House and adjacent to the U.S. Treasury Department.

Just three blocks from our lunch destination we were halted in our limousine as President Obama was coming down Pennsylvania Avenue in his Cadillac motorcade known as "The Beast" adorned with the Secret Service installed red and blue lights blaring and motorcycles and armored cars accompanied by no less than a hundred agents. Once again, to say it was surreal was an understatement. By God's grace and Meadowlark's generosity I am sitting in his limo while we are watching the leader of the free world drive by in his.

Being both in the Nation's Capital and literally almost born inside the Capitol Building I was fortunate to be listen in person and be in the presence of six U.S. Presidents and shook hands with three by my 35th birthday. What was even more surreal is at that moment, at that intersection, in two respective limousines just feet away for a nanosecond we were connected. President Obama wrote Meadowlark's foreword and I was blessed to as well because of

God above and the man beside me in the car. Once again, regardless if paupers to Presidents they all had an affinity for the ambassador of basketball and Globetrotter of JOY.

We walked into the restaurant and they are used to political power but when Meadowlark walked in it was something else. They graciously seated us in a comfortable location and we had a time! Later that afternoon, we watched some college football together on television only to race off in the limo towards an event he was doing that night at Columbia University. He asked me to accompany him and I assisted with his merchandise table and had a wonderful dinner among some distinguished guests and as always, he was stellar with his remarks.

Most folks associated us together as a team but one asked if I were an aide to him? The funny thing was I had been an aide to a Member of Congress, all 100 United States Senators, Vice President when appointed by the Senate Sergeant at Arms in April 1995, to be a bi-partisan figure on the floor and also an aide to the Governor of Maryland in 2000-2001. In that brief moment it dawned on me that I was both a friend but also occasional aide to Meadowlark. With his last name, Lemon it just stuck and we created LEMON aide.

It's true when life hands you LEMONs, get up and make lemonade! And that is exactly what we did! After another action packed weekend in Washington, D.C. he flew back out of town but before he left we did get to spend some quality time with his daughter who works at the Pentagon. She is also an American hero in her own right and regardless how many stars are on one's epaulettes, when Meadowlark walked down the hall they all stopped to salute him. When you realize you humbly carry greatness then greatness carries you to places of honor.

To this day, whenever, Meadowlark and I catch up whether by phone or in person it's like we never missed a beat. Then again when you have as much rhythm as that brother (Lark) you cannot help but bounce to the music.

Since leaving my Capitol Hill job on July 27, 2007, I speak up to 200 dates per year counting radio and television appearances. You cannot lose when you think to help others. One afternoon nearly three years ago, I was driving in my hometown and for the strangest reason all I could think of was St. Louis,

Missouri. Anyone who is self employed or travels across the Country as an artist or speaker knows firsthand not only how grueling it can be to travel but also how much faith and fortitude it takes to stay on the road "by faith."

Knowing that Meadowlark is ideal for schools, corporate events and church services I just thought I should be proactive to try to open a door for him. Initially, it was tempting to think that since he is known around the Globe by his first name he probably doesn't need any help why bother or would it be embarrassing to try to help. Actually, I have found we all need help. Secondly, we find nothing like the value of a referral and thirdly, many may have either thought he was inactive, cost too much to come or worse, deceased. Many do think "out of sight – out of mind."

God had blessed me to be in a few major cities across the Country but all I could think of was St. Louis. I called Meadowlark and he answered in his deep voice: "Brother Frank!" I smiled and said: "Sir, I don't know why and I may be wrong for calling and don't mean to inconvenience you but if you ever find yourself back in St. Louis let me know because I have two or three clergy friends that would love to have you minister to their congregation." He thanked me for the call and he was grateful for the Kingdom connection and assured me he would be back in touch.

Not long afterwards, true to his word he had his wife Dr. Cynthia Lemon call me out of the blue and she said, "Frank, my husband, Meadowlark and I are so grateful for all you have done to help him and he wants to help you." I said: "Dr. Lemon, you both already have because I can't believe we have grown as friends. It is my honor." She said: "It was interesting you mentioned St. Louis because Meadowlark is already scheduled to be there in less than two months. I can't accompany him on this trip but he wants to know if you will meet him there?"

In previous chapters you may recall me hearing theme songs in my head regardless, if "Moving on Up" from the Jefferson's or "I'm a Soul Man" by the Blues Brothers but now I remember hearing some tune as a child "Meet Me in Saint Louie." Not asking why, I said "Yes Ma'am!" She went on to explain that Meadowlark serves on the board of Major League Baseball great Albert Pujols' Foundation for children with Down Syndrome and his annual gala was going to be at a five star hotel in downtown St Louis. She then said, "Since I cannot make the dinner, you get to be his date" and we are going to pay for your airfare.

Then if that wasn't enough she said: "Meadowlark wants you to introduce him at all three churches you arrange for him to speak in Missouri and Illinois." Again, the doors you open for others God may open for you. The baseball playoffs were well under way and I began to watch more than ever with anticipation following Albert's season. The next month, the St. Louis Cardinals won the World Series and just three weeks later I would have the high honor to accompany arguably one of basketball's greatest players to be introduced to one of baseball's present day greatest players.

We got a wonderful picture of the three us, Meadowlark on the left, Albert in the middle and me, the glorified goofball to the right. Forrest Gump would have fit right in! At the dinner that night were also baseball icons, Don Mattingly "Mr. Baseball," Lou Brock and if that wasn't enough who rolled up in a wheelchair but none other than 91- year-old Stan "The Man" Musial. I didn't trouble him for a picture but he shook my hand and all I could think of was my father who I wished could have been there that night. He would have loved it!

This was my father's generation and his heroes and I wish I could have moved Heaven and Earth to make this moment possible. Knowing the greats are gracious but not wanting to look desperate or ungrateful to Meadowlark because when you are with the best you don't want to bypass anyone in the process. I was Meadowlark's guest and it was by God's grace that I was befriended by him. Later that evening, I caught up with Don Mattingly and asked him if I could get an autograph for my father and he scribbled his autograph on a brand new baseball. No doubt, as I gingerly placed it in a protective bag I knew once again I was "carrying greatness."

Albert Pujols gave me a gorgeous hand signed picture of him with the Cardinals that I will cherish forever and a brand new $250 iPod. How many people get a gift from a World Series winner two weeks before Christmas? Some say it is wrong to repackage a gift but I didn't see any harm in giving my wife, Ruth that musical play box. Plus, we live completely "by faith" and just because one is a preacher who occasionally speaks on television doesn't mean we have the finances of a televangelist. Plus, I was trying to think of others more than of myself. It was God's grace and this mindset that opened these doors to begin with.

Just two months before, I spent two hours in Richmond, VA with baseball icon, Pete Rose and he graciously signed a baseball and autographed a bat that I made clear I wanted to present for my father. Some collect to sell but mostly I have found it more fun to give. That night, I was blessed to take a picture with Pete and that was enough for me. In my heart, I believe we need to shine during every door God opens for us but share the wealth and experiences with others. We all win when we promote others.

That night was an unforgettable evening in St. Louis and just like the Winston-Salem week with one of God's greatest generals I would have missed St. Louis if I didn't think out of the box, promote others and have faith to follow through. Less than a week later, Albert Pujols surprised everyone and signed with the Angels in California for a $253 Million contract. Many fans were sad and shocked but I knew that Christian brother was going to shine a Light wherever he went. The Bible notes, "Whatever your hand finds to do, make sure you do it for His glory." It was getting late and the crowd was beginning to clear out and Meadowlark and I had a very busy next two days.

The very next morning we had two church services in Missouri and another one that night at a mega church in Illinois. It was my honor to chaperone him, introduce and assist him with merchandise at both churches in the morning. God showed up, the crowd went wild and he shined like a million lights flicking for the Gospel's glory. When you know and love The Light you cannot help but beam bright. We went to a steak house in Missouri with our dear friend, Ronnie Dean "The Preaching Machine." He has preached over 8,000 sermons in his life and his nickname is "The Raven," They say "birds of a feather flock together" and now we have Meadowlark, The Raven and Parakeet (me) all dining at the same time in the 'Show Me' state of Missouri.

When we walked in it was as if all eyes were on us but I knew it wasn't because I now knew better. All eyes were on him but I was honored to be in the same state, room and vicinity. God had allowed me to be around greatness and it was not only deposited in me but next to me. Actually all around me because God doesn't make any junk. Just because some folks don't believe in

God doesn't mean that God ceases to believe in them! The Creator of the world sees everyone with love and we win when walk and talk with God.

Meadowlark, The Raven and I found a seat and folks politely came by like a popular drive in restaurant one by one wanting to say hi, thanks for the memories, may I get a picture or will you sign my napkin? He graciously accommodated them all but never failed to remember to honor those who 'carried' him that day.

One of the greatest attributes is not just his charm, charisma or countless credentials but I have seen him up close and personal what many have not. He is loyal all day long. For starters, regarding his loyalty, he didn't ask me to introduce him that night which is an honor but he said, "Brother Frank, I want you to preach for fifteen minutes before you introduce me before I get up." He knew to dance with the one he went with at the prom and he didn't owe me a thing but he knew life and leadership is a team effort. He didn't dominate in basketball by being selfish on the hardwood and he wasn't about to drop the ball in ministry.

The event went so well that the pastor, who was a dear friend of mine, told me before the service started he would like to bring me back to preach revival at their awesome church in Illinois. Ironically, if I didn't try to help a friend out in St. Louis I may have never made it back down the road. Since then, I have been back four times in two years.

Another element of Meadowlark's loyalty is that night after leaving that church service in the "land of Lincoln" while dining at Steak and Shake. We were enjoying a milkshake when another local pastor approached our table and wanted to say "hi." The back story is Ronnie is beloved all around that part of the Country but some folks are too small to compliment. He didn't want to fellowship with Ronnie previously but when he is now seen dining with one of the most famous people in the world he comes up like they are long, lost friends.

The Preaching Machine (Ronnie) took the high road and still introduced the icon and his personal friend to the pastor. For the record, even pastors are human and now for a brief moment by God's grace and Ronnie's generosity forgot the past and enabled the man who had hurt him to now have time in the sun despite late in the evening with his childhood hero. Unfortunately, this minister in Missouri failed again. If it were not enough that Ronnie forgot the past, this clergy failed in the present and had the audacity to try to take a cheap shot at Ronnie while in the presence of Meadowlark. Our dear friend, Lark may have been born at night but not last night and he graciously shot down the minister's rebuke and the pastor shot himself in the foot because their conversation was now over. It was just like how it started when we walked in just God, Meadowlark, Ronnie and me and that was actually a good place to be.

We finished our meal and headed back towards the hotel and Meadowlark once again invited us to come in and watch football with him. Never once did I take those precious moments together for granted because life is short and I never knew when it may be the last. As long as I live, I will never forget what transpired next. We were watching the remainder of a Sunday evening NFL game in the hotel and it was late in the third quarter and Tim Tebow was the quarterback for the Denver Broncos.

Tebow was marching his team down the field with great precision and Meadowlark was cheering for him. With every completed pass, first down or exciting play his chants for the white guy on the screen grew louder. Tebow was on fire and Meadowlark was beside himself and he was clapping his hands at every completed pass.

I'm not the smartest person on the planet but I could clearly see something. Meadowlark was beside himself, lost in the moment cheering for another brother. It hit me that I was now having more fun watching him cheer for Tebow than watching the game itself. I will go to my grave that at that moment, Meadowlark was having more fun cheering for Tebow than Tim was having leading his team to victory. Plus, here is one of the greatest athletes of all time cheering for the younger generation. Even more special was the fact not that this Hall of Fame basketball icon who was already accomplished in his own right was cheering for an up and comer who hadn't even won the Big Game yet. What was more profound is the fact that Meadowlark as a colored athlete faced such hostility and hatred among others in the past despite bringing JOY to millions and he's now presently pushing, pulling and praying for a white kid to not only do well but to WIN!

Tebow was on a roll and the next thing I know Meadowlark in his late 70's is now on the bed! He's not only on the bed but clapping his hands like a seal and jumping up and down on the hotel bed going crazy rooting for Tebow. I have seen a few things in life but that will be burned in my memory until God calls me Home. At that moment, I wish every person in the world could see what I witnessed with my own eyes but this brother not only loved God, the game or sports but wanted this guy (Tebow) to be successful. God showed me years ago that "winners are wonderful but it's the wannabe you have to watch out for!" Those who have been to the mountain can compliment at the drop of a hat to wish another well without feeling threatened. The rest only know complaint, curse words or criticism.

I thought I admired Meadowlark for the iconic American flag shorts, his half court hook shot or for bringing JOY to millions. The truth is, I admire him far more as the minister he is in public and the class act he is in private. He really is the genuine article. After connecting Ronnie and Meadowlark together who would have guessed but that "Dynamic Duo" went on to do 75 events together in multiple states. It never ceases to fail that Meadowlark will call me just to check in and he always calls on Christmas Day or Easter. The guy known around the globe still has time to reach out to an individual and yes, the greats are gracious.

My fourth grade friend, Joe is the man. I look forward to reuniting with him soon and all is forgiven. Truth be told, I never got that Harlem Globetrotter jersey but I got so much more. Who would have ever thought that I would have the privilege to grow as friends with Meadowlark? The replica jersey was temporal but our friendship is eternal. The jersey would have been lost but I found a lifelong friend with the living legend. In fourth grade when the jersey never came, as a freckle-faced kid, I felt I was wrongfully dealt lemons but God knew better and as an adult, by God's grace, we made LEMON aide.

CHAPTER SEVEN

"NO LONGER RUTH-LESS"

During the darkest days of my life the Lord gave me a vision. Dr. Adrian Rogers said,

"Never doubt in the dark what the Lord showed you in the light." God revealed to me that I would marry a woman with olive skin, long dark hair and she would be slightly older than me. This woman would have an exotic look opposed to the "girl next door" and despite her curves without question her values would walk the straight and narrow and love God as much as me.

He even gave me a glimpse of the wedding dress she would wear and would you believe she wore the same one I had in my mind. I may have been a fish out of water but she was the miracle and mermaid of my dreams. I put out a fleece to the Lord and we had a budget like most couples and our goal wasn't to spend tens of thousands on a wedding like too many but not a dime on the marriage. We were in it for the long haul and death do us part was not rhetoric but a reality in our relationship.

Our first date was in February 2007, and our third date was Valentines' Day. Some suggest don't move too fast, or look desperate, but when you know – you know! Ruth and I got engaged after a scenic dinner date on a cruise that went up the Potomac River and we watched the magnificent monuments in Washington, D.C. When the boat docked we got back to Alexandria, VA and I drove to the Lincoln Memorial and we walked up the iconic steps and visited President Abraham Lincoln and saw the amazing view of the National Mall. We descended down the steps halfway and about the exact spot that Dr.

Martin Luther King, Jr. gave the famous "I Have a Dream" speech is where I intended to propose to Ruth.

No joke, I began to get a tad nervous. I have always been one to speak to crowds in my sleep but if it were someone (just one) I actually have a harder time communicating. Apparently, I was so nervous that it was apparent to a man walking with his wife accompanying a camera and he could see something was getting ready to go down. Now with a bystander watching and paparazzi taking pictures I asked Elda Ruth Salmeron to marry me with God above, President Lincoln looking from behind with the National Mall and our future in front. By God's grace, she said "YES!"

As I began to look for a church to get married we decided on July 2007 (same year). Our first date was in February 12, 2007, and married just a few months later. Here is where the fleece came in even before proposing. I knew that July would be a tough time to have a wedding on such short notice but I also knew that "with God ALL things are possible." I knew we needed a couple things to fall into place before asking Ruth's hand in marriage.

With time ticking, I needed to find a church, reception hall and see if my Best Man would be available. These three may not seem like much to you but when time is of the essence and we wanted to get married on one of the most booked days in modern memory for a wedding and lastly, when you speak upwards to 200 dates per year and your best man travels even more than you, getting everyone on board would not be a minor but major miracle!

Previously, I had officiated a wedding and preached twice at a beautiful church just miles from our home in Southern Maryland. Victory Chapel was still fairly new and absolutely gorgeous! Immediately, I called the church secretary and told her I was hoping to get married the second Saturday in July and she said: "Rev. Shelton, that Saturday will be hard to get and we already have a wedding scheduled earlier that day but for you I have a feeling that God will work it out!" I won't mislead you, I was down when she said "booked" already but curious and grateful she was confident that God would work it out for me and her assurance gave me peace. Ironically, she ministered to me. She called back with a laugh and said: "Minister Shelton, I told you God would work it out. The pastor just said you can have the church for an afternoon wedding!" PRAISE THE LORD!!

We had one down and two more to go (reception hall and Best Man) because this would be the trifecta to see if this was really of the Lord. Ruth and I visited the beautiful Tantallon Golf Course Country Club overlooking the Potomac River near Washington, D.C. It is a gorgeous Georgian Colonial mansion with stately columns and ideal to host our family and friends.

What were the odds? When I contacted the coordinator to see about pricing and availability who answered the phone but Ronnie Rufner, a high school classmate whom I had not spoken to in nearly two decades! They also had a wedding scheduled that day but he said if we would wait until five in the evening he could clean it up and accommodate us for our wedding. God provided the miracle and Ronnie and his team worked their "magic" and now we were two for two!

Ruth and I had lunch that afternoon at the country club after meeting with Ronnie but the clock was ticking because it was just a few months prior to our wedding. We were both excited and optimistic that God would work it out for my buddy, Sam to be present as my Best Man. I called him in Chicago and asked him to check his calendar and he said, "Congrats Frank, but I must be honest I am slammed this entire summer with speaking and traveling and not certain I can make it. Let me check my calendar and I will call you first of the week." When he called back he replied: "I checked and the only weekend I have available is July 7, 2007." The good news is that was the very date of our wedding, 07-07-07.

Those numbers are Biblical and represent perfection and restoration. We serve an on-time God and He does all things well. Plus, He is never in a hurry but ALWAYS on time! Dr. Adrian Rogers was right, "never doubt in the dark what the Lord showed you in the light." Ruth and I were married among family and friends and the wedding was officiated by our dear friend and pastor, Rev. Marvin Harris. The scenery was gorgeous and my wife looked flawless. The Lord put it all together not just in the wedding but the miracle of our marriage.

That evening when we arrived at our hotel we had an early morning flight to Cancun, Mexico for our honeymoon! Another gift from God is that a precious pastor friend of Ruth felt led to pay for our airfare and accommodations in Mexico as a gift! That evening as I stood at the hotel door I put our bags down, opened the door and picked up my wife. I looked at this beautiful bombshell that God had entrusted me and picked her up and carried her into our room. Without question, at that very moment I knew I was carrying greatness. Like any valuable present, it is mandatory to handle with care.

When my children Hannah Grace and Andrew Lincoln were born I was blessed both times to be in the hospital delivery room. Hannah was born on April 30, 2000 and Andrew was born on January 20, 2009. He was born the same exact day President Obama was inaugurated and I was born President's Day Weekend, February 20, 1972. As the 44th President was "coming in" our baby boy, Andrew was "coming out."

As if it were yesterday, I recall being ushered into the delivery room and was given surgical gloves and had the high honor to catch my daughter, Hannah as she was birthed. Over the years, I have held innumerable objects, grabbed countless boxes and had a million and one things in my hands in four decades of life. As our baby was closer to being born my mind raced when as a youth when I played sports I could see in the highlight reel of my life with a fresh focus the times I made a one hand catch in football or an amazing grab in baseball or grabbed a rebound off the glass that the entire gym erupted in delight but also remembered the time I dropped the ball and sand slipped through my fingers at the beach. With the clocking ticking and the baby almost here I prayed a silent prayer with my eyes wide open that God wouldn't let me drop the ball (baby) now.

Never before had I been so focused and nothing else in the world mattered in that moment. My wife did all the work and all I needed to do was hold on for dear life, actually both of our lives; Hannah's and mine. I knew that she was a child and not a choice and even John the Baptist was alive enough to stand when Jesus was in both the womb and room.

The instant I held Hannah for the first time I knew I was holding something special. It was greater than Beethoven's Best and more valuable than all the riches of Egypt. She was birthed in love and loaned from Heaven and immediately I know that even being "slow" I was holding greatness. When taking our children in and out of the car seat I knew I was holding greatness. Some may say, "Frank, relax every parent feels that way!" With nearly sixty million abortions I wish I were wrong. Children are a gift from God and it is a huge privilege to be a parent. By God's grace, I didn't drop her at Southern Maryland Hospital and will never let go. However, I have learned that with all gifts that we are really just a custodian. They belong to God and a form of worship is having our hands and palms opened wide lifting towards Heaven. I have also had to learn that we are to hold our children close but also like a bicycle with training wheel there comes a time when we have to let them go after giving them to God. His nail scarred hands are much safer and stronger than ours,

The same is true with a gift. It is like a book on loan from the local library. We don't really own it but we are entrusted with it temporarily and we have a huge fine to pay if we don't care or misplace it on our watch. Yes, we must develop our gifts and protect it, share it but if we hoard it then we all lose. Again, we can carry or bury greatness. With our children today, we pray daily (sometimes hourly) for them and ask that God will guide us all as we follow Him. It has been said, "You will never lose your footing when you have been on your knees.

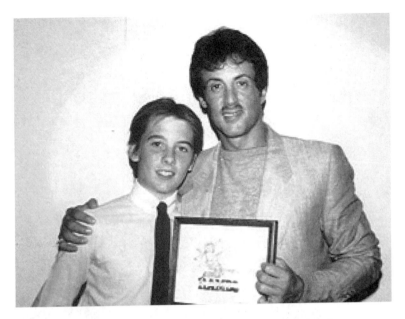

Frank (age 13) & Sly Stallone - Hollywood, CA (1985)

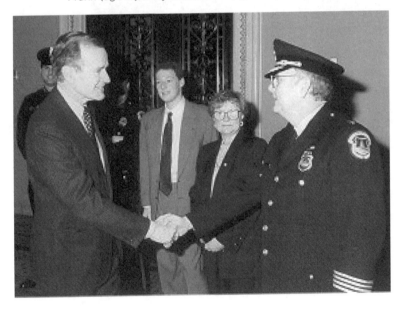

Dad & Pres George H.W. Bush - Wash DC (1992)

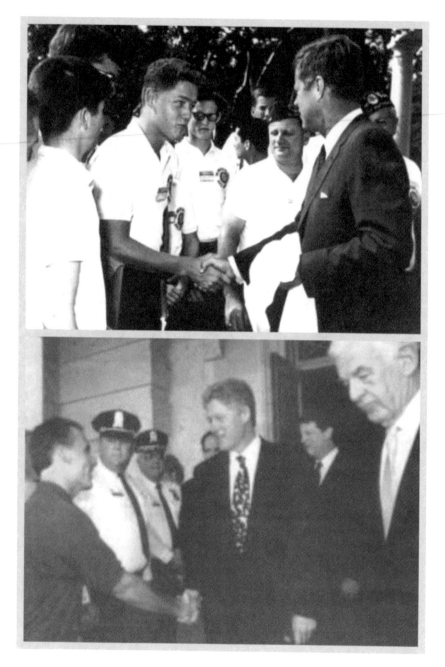

JFK & Bill Clinton (1963) & Frank & Pres Clinton (1993)

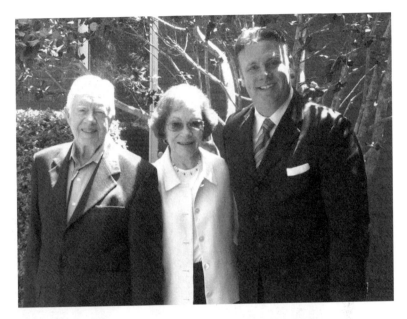

Frank & Pres Jimmy Carter - Plains, GA (2013)

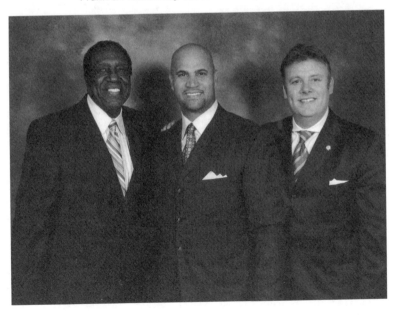

Meadowlark Lemon & Albert Pujols - St Louis, MO (2011)

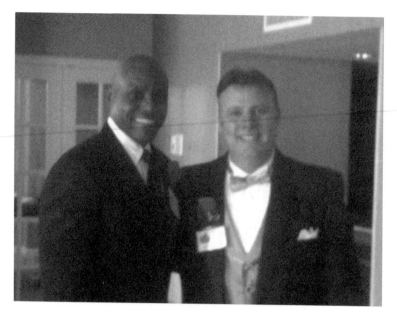

Olympian Carl Lewis - Dallas, TX (2011)

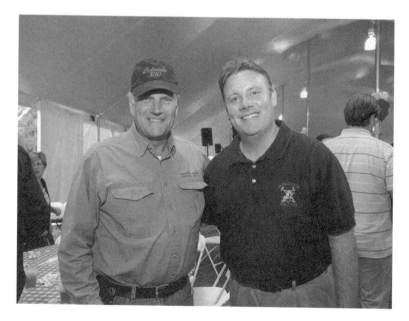

Rev Franklin Graham - Boone, NC (2011)

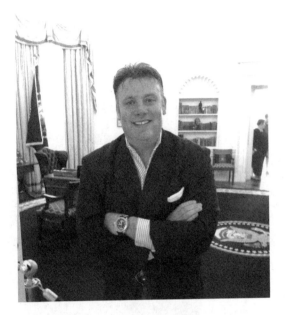

Frank at the Oval Office

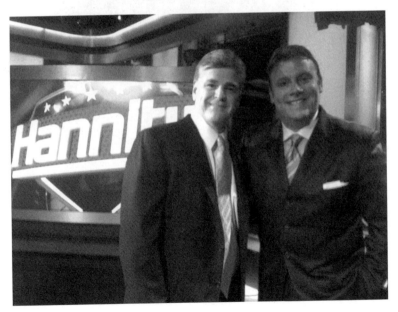

Sean HANNITY - New York City (2014)

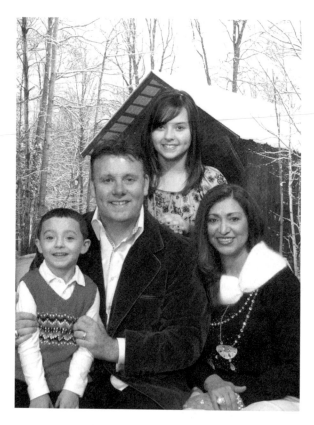

Shelton Family - CHRISTmas

CHAPTER EIGHT

KING OF A NATION

General George Washington was invited and even implored to become king and at the height of his honor showed humility. He uttered the words that we all needed but not everyone at the time wanted. He said, "There will be no king but King Jesus!" His faith became the foundation and framework for our young nation and out of the gate a nation couldn't settle for anyone because mediocrity was not an option. Anyone could have derailed or destroyed the great experiment called America.

From that day forward, the presidency would be an institution not an individual and future presidents would be the closest to a king we would ever have in the present. History remembers powerful presidents but often over looks common people. We fail to see the mundane standing next to magnificent but God and the "greats" don't.

President Abraham Lincoln was correct when he said, "God must have loved so many ordinary people because He made so many of us." I also think it's cool that the Commander-in-Chief would consider himself one of the mundane. Yes, the greats are gracious. Perhaps that is just another reason why he reached the mountain top. President Lincoln's image is on both the five dollar bill and penny. For years, I was offended that someone of his stature would be reduced to our entry level currency but it dawned on me that he was great because he was accessible to all. Both commoners and high society touched him and could learn from him. He wasn't an isolated elitist but, like my Lord, accessible, approachable and available to all. He didn't come for the few but for the masses and he loved people and people loved him.

We all know him to be our sixteenth president but his personal losses shaped him long before political success. He failed privately before he fought for freedom publicly and he was weary individually long before winning the war on slavery collectively. He knew the scorn of rejection and didn't take promotion for granted. Elisabeth and Mary both were rejected in private before birthing greatness in public. If you have never lost you are not prepared to win. Lincoln's rejection enabled him to offer acceptance to so many and he treated everyone with class and courtesy. Whether speaking to a shackled slave or to his Secretary of State, he saw both with innate value. He was a builder of men not a wrecking ball for mankind.

He knew dark nights and deep depression intimately but was living proof that light shines bright in the deepest well and darkest backdrops. Jewelers intentionally place their brightest diamonds on a black setting to allow their true beauty to shine and illuminate. Lincoln had lost repeatedly for local office before reaching the pinnacle of political power. Those very scars along the way shaped the man to be in a better position and thus a better person to lead the nation. We love him not because he went undefeated but he was unrelenting in accomplishing not only broad goals but noble causes to make us a better country.

Lincoln had lost a fiancé to death and that almost destroyed him. Losing any election is devastating but losing almost a dozen should have derailed him. He knew it gets quiet if you quit and patriotism, perseverance and public service were the inner callings that compelled him as he steered us.

Some considered him strange and aloof and others went as far to call him square. However, America needed someone square to display true leadership in an office that today happens to be Oval. He was the right man, at the right time for the task at hand and he not only led the people but truly loved them. He was not a dictator but a country lawyer that had a great gift to read people and was well read himself. He was a quick study and equipped with an amazing gift to inject humor that helped break barriers and build trust with friends and foe alike.

He was self deprecating and perhaps that is another reason why we honor him so. He took his work seriously but not himself as much. He knew that public service was a noble calling and he was selfless not selfish. When he arrived at The White House he had to come in under the radar. He found no honeymoon experience after being inaugurated and the Washington elite thought the backwoods lawyer was outdated. He was gangly and walked awkwardly and aesthetically was not much to look at. He was tall and rugged but stood head and shoulders above most, not just in height but also in honor.

Every good leader knows timing is everything. He wasn't out to make history; history was making him, but he never bent under pressure. He didn't break but blessed us all in the process. Lincoln made friends easily and recalled names like very few and he made everyone feel important. Those who endure the deepest depression make the lasting impressions and he was no exception.

He was not only for the people but was also one of them. At times he was known personally to answer the front door of the Executive Mansion. One of the great attributes of any leader and certainly of Lincoln was that he listened. Whether he was listening to his spouse, senators, soldiers, staff or a slave, he made each feel important. Sadly, in our social media world of today that kind of rare respect is all but gone.

Perhaps this combination made for the perfect marriage between two totally different individuals brewing. You may recall in a previous chapter, Cup of Joe, we'll pull up a seat and feast at the table with a plate of presidential friendship. In one corner we find arguably the most beloved Commander-in-Chief in history (Lincoln) and in another we find a cop. One is President of the Country and the other a policeman in the city. It was said at President John F. Kennedy's funeral that several of the pallbearers were Secret Service agents. After you spent quality time with someone they become an extension of the family. It is also appropriate that after just passing the 50th anniversary of President Kennedy's assassination in November of last year the irony is newsmen were called on to be pallbearers at Lee Harvey Oswald's funeral because he didn't even have six friends to carry his casket. For decades, I have said, "Winners are wonderful but it is the wannabe you have to watch out for."

President Lincoln's popularity was at an all time low. The polls were down, morale was bleak and the presidential honeymoon never started for him.

Truthfully, his marriage resembled a mirage and his days in his office included dark nights which didn't help with his bouts with depression. Perhaps with his public leadership came private loneliness. His wife wanted little to do with him while grieving in her own way over the death of their son and being isolated in Washington's ivory tower didn't help the situation. Ironically, the one dominated by darkness in the day helped light the way in the darkest nights of our country. Perhaps even more poignant was the irony that the one who carried and rallied the masses often felt all alone.

He knew power but also pain and quite possibly what he needed most was fellowship. Enter D.C. policeman Joseph Gales who was assigned to The White House. While working overtime, he became friendly with President Lincoln. On occasion, the two of them would cross paths and small talk at both the Executive Mansion and en route to an event.

Quite a combination, you have heard of "An Officer and a Gentleman" but a century and a half before we find a President and policeman. No doubt, Lincoln was definitely a gentleman. Long before Gere made it big in Hollywood we have Gales a century earlier in the White House. Their friendship grew and it was once written that President Lincoln signed a special order excluding Joseph Gales from military duty during the Civil War so he could remain in his and Mrs. Lincoln's service at the White House.

If you knew anything about Joseph's family is that they are honest, hardworking and full of humor. They are known to constantly have a joke and quick wit to all whom they meet and their service to God and Country earned them the respect of their peers and made countless friends from janitors to executives.

God has an uncanny way of strategically placing His children in the path of both the prominent and poor. With the President's poll numbers declining and his wife constantly whining perhaps this friendly cop was a shining a light of friendship and gift of fellowship. As the Civil War raged and body count of the war rose, the circles under his eyes grew darker and the weight of the world became unbearable on his shoulders. The President aptly noted, "At times, I had nowhere else to turn but to God on my knees."

Great leaders know the value of time and they realize tomorrow is not guaranteed. Lincoln despite being President most likely today would not have adorned a Rolex "Presidential" watch. A genuine Rolex second hand is unlike any other because it doesn't hesitate and our sixteenth president would have probably related more to the hour glass because it would remind him and us all that eventually time will run out.

Sometimes a lack of urgency leads to catastrophe and Lincoln definitely knew time was short. I cannot help but think that perhaps on many of those sleepless nights the President would pace the lonely halls of power and pause to speak to the hired help, policemen on patrol and his friend who happened to be a cop, Joseph Gales.

President Lincoln, despite great odds, accomplished so much in such a short period of time. He knew in life you can do two things, either invest time or waste it. He knew that his clock was ticking and he worked continuously. He knew that the time he had as president would be short but I am convinced that he knew his life would be shorter. With no time to spare, he helped free the slaves, had the motto "In God We Trust" engraved on our currency, implemented the National Day of Prayer and to this day is still the most quoted American in history. He built bridges not walls and he was civil to even those that despised him.

As I write this chapter in November 2013, we are just three days away from the 150th anniversary of President Lincoln making Thanksgiving a national holiday. In November 1863, the president proclaimed that day and asked the nation that all Americans repent of their perversity. That takes boldness and that is true leadership. We always ask for God to bless America and He has, but the better route would be that we, as Americans, bless God.

Today, while speaking and preaching across America, I have the honor to be a volunteer White House Press Correspondent with Intermountain Christian News and attend briefings at the James S. Brady Room in the West Wing. Dr. Anthony Harper, Editor of the Christian Newspaper has said in private and publicly at The White House that we should return to the request of President Lincoln for a national repentance. True repentance leads to revival and regardless of your political persuasion, we should pray for our current President and his family. The job load is immense and the stakes are enormous and I would encourage you to write a letter to your Members of Congress and local politicians to let them know you are praying for them and that God will guide their effort, action and attitude. President Ronald Reagan said, "If we ever cease to be one nation under God we will become a nation gone under."

Yes, for decades many Americans and elected leaders celebrated Thanksgiving but it didn't become a national holiday until President Lincoln. In 1621, Governor William Bradford of the Plymouth Colony, paused and celebrated with the Pilgrims after they survived that first harsh winter in America. Samuel Adams, during the Second Continental Congress, did the same. Despite not being a religious person, The Honorable Thomas Jefferson along with over a thousand others also celebrated a day of giving thanks, but it wasn't until a woman named Hale pleaded with politicians for two decades that Lincoln made it official. Similar to my ancestor and his crew planting the Cherry Blossoms, perseverance pays off.

It is important to note that President Lincoln had just given his life to Christ after seeing the blood bath, carnage and gore at Gettysburg. With each step on the sacred soil and as blood and mud squashed beneath his boots he couldn't help on Earth to realize he needed help from above. President Lincoln knew that despite the closest to a royalty America will ever have he still needed assistance and a personal relationship with the God of the Universe. Humility comes before honor and we are humbled to realize that Heaven sent the Son of God to bleed on our behalf and became the payment from the penalty of sin that had plagued us down. Only Jesus, the Living Water, could give His rich, red blood to wash our muddy sins as white as new fallen snow. That conversion to Christ compelled him to free the slaves not only because he knew now that God created all men equal but if the God of the universe had freed him personally he could do nothing less than free all corporately. All of us are shackled by sin and bound by the fall of man as a result of Adam and Eve's sin, but Christ sets the captives free and extends pardon to us by accepting His propitiation as the payment for our sins.

We are saved by grace and through faith (Ephesians 2:8-9). Lincoln knew loss, leadership and loneliness but now knew personally the Lord. He knew that like Christ his time would be cut short and because he lived a legacy he would leave a legacy. For decades it was said if the president asked you to do something you do it but crowds are fickle and outside of God above and a few friends beside him, he probably felt alone.

While vacationing in Gettysburg with my family in 2010, I recall reading that President Lincoln had invited no less than a dozen people to be his guests along with his wife, Mary Todd to watch "Our American Cousin" at Ford's Theater. All of them turned him down save for Henry Rathbone and Clara Harris. Once again, the obvious isn't obvious and leadership is lovely but comes with a lonely price tag.

I often wonder what kind of conversation that the cop from Washington had with the world's most powerful person. Did he share one of his corny jokes with the Commander in Chief? Did he make the president laugh so hard that when his belly buckled gasping for air because of the much needed humor did his iconic stove top hat fall unto the floor? It was noted the president often hid his speech inside his hat so when folks said "the president speaks from the top of his head" they were not kidding. If those notes fell to the ground I would bet a year's wages that it was the policeman who bent down to pick them up. President Lincoln did more than speak from the top of his head but the bottom of his heart and that is why he is endeared to millions.

Even then, during the day festivities at the White House were crazy. The President probably could only give a glance or occasional wink to one of his favorite policemen. Other times, without saying a word maybe a wave or a quick pat on the back because now knowing he personally dealt privately with depression he was the consummate cheerleader in public. Perhaps "Encourager in Chief" was more fitting for Lincoln but because he humbly encouraged he was worthy to lead all those under his command.

If he wasn't talking with the hired help or the security working midnight Lincoln could be found doing two things. Sadly, his wife was not much of a comfort and that forced him to pray more than ever. He would petition God in prayer for wisdom, strength and friendship and his ever present pocket watch reminded him repeatedly like the rhythms of life could hear each tick clearer and louder. The president knew his days were numbered and with God's help he was going to die living make each day count.

The pressure of the presidency mounted on his shoulders more than ever and the days were long and nights longer. It is ironic and borderline tragic that the most powerful person on the planet couldn't rally his own spouse to support him personally or politicians of his own party at times to follow him professionally. God above and his acquaintance, Joseph the cop below probably offered the rare solace that he needed.

His popularity had plummeted but his mission was much greater than fame. His goal was not even that his name would be remembered but he had a keen sense that doing right is greater than possessing military might. With each passing day it was as if the clock that once chimed so loud was beginning to tick low. His entire life, especially en route to the presidency knew constantly that time was not his friend but a foe he had to deal with daily. The ticks of his proverbial life clock seemed to pass like a race horse out the gate. He accomplished more with less and would eventually die leaving us with more than we have ever had personally or as a Country.

Lincoln at this juncture related more to an hour glass than his beloved pocket watch. The statesman studied the sand in the hour glass more than ever because he knew his time was about up. It was reported that President Abraham Lincoln when leaving the White House would always say "see you later" to his friends, family and staff on the way out but on this night en route to the theater he said, "good bye." Like Elvis, with a tip of his trademark hat and a slight twinkle in his eye he left the building.

They arrived at Ford's Theater to a capacity crowd and everyone was enjoying themselves at a night on the town. As the play progressed, a Maryland native and renowned actor, John Wilkes Booth was in the house. He was the ideal assassin because he had celebrity and access. The actor was fuming and he had one thing on his mind: to execute the President. Almost a century later, Oswald hadn't done anything and in acting circles but the famed Booth had accomplished almost everything. Sadly, both had gifts but used them for harm and not to help. Those who hurt often do hurtful things.

Just five days before General Robert E. Lee surrendered his army at

Appomattox Court House, VA and that act ended the Civil War. On Good Friday, April 14, 1865 the off duty actor Booth was not acting and his sole mission was to kill the Commander- in- Chief. His plot was not stopping with Lincoln but he wanted to throw the U.S. government into disarray by also plotting to assassinate Vice President Johnson and Secretary of State William Seward. For a man who lived at theater he was not playing around.

While the President and his wife watched the performance above the stage in a private box it was appropriate that Lincolns are seated and conversing with a young Army officer named Rathbone and his fiancé. Here we find the most powerful man in the world and commander of every general on down and yet Lincoln is side by side enjoying the company of an entry level officer. To Lincoln, he saw value not in titles but in their character and potential. He deemed character of more worth than credentials or cash and perhaps that symbolizes the friendship with the President and a policeman named Joseph Gales. Plus, the president who found salvation and a relationship with Christ knew that at the foot of the cross the ground is level.

Secure people don't need prominent people of position or power around them to feel important. Actually, they gravitate towards those who could use encouragement and mentoring. On this night, the man who knew depression well was also known to bring comic relief to others. The presidential delegation was in a jovial mood and even laughed during the play.

Approximately at 10:15 PM EST, John Wilkes Booth slipped into the presidential box and fired his personal .44 caliber Derringer in the back of Lincoln's head. Officer Rathbone rushed towards Booth but was stabbed by the actor in the shoulder and he jumped to the stage shouting "*Sic semper tyrannis!*" Translating the State of Virginia motto – "Thus ever to tyrants!"

The crowd thought that it was part of the play as if the leading man of that era was in a cameo. However, the shrill from the First Lady eliminated that thought immediately. The crowd roared, the President groaned and the play was over. If only they were still acting!

After hearing Mrs. Lincoln's screams, a 23- year-old doctor who was in attendance was beckoned to attend to the bleeding President. Once again, we find novices at the scene and around the President in life and now imminent death. Again, that is why he is on our penny because true leadership is accessible and approachable. Lincoln embodied that trait and he was to be touched by all not just the elite few. The man who gave his best believed in others too and now a soldier with fresh blood from Booth's stab and a young doctor is doing his best to stop the President from bleeding to death.

As Dr. Charles Reade desperately attended to the President the crowd was in complete pandemonium. The First Lady and almost everyone else resembled the state of the President – they are in shock. Despite breaking his leg when jumping off the balcony, Booth was still able to exit the theater and escape on horseback from Washington heading to his native Maryland.

We do find some startling similarity between the two assassins. Oswald didn't have an escape plan but Booth did. Booth used a small gun and Oswald used a big rifle but darn if both of them shot their target in the head and both having ties to a theater. Oswald was arrested in a theater in downtown Dallas after shooting Kennedy and Booth performed his worse act at Ford's Theater and both were successful in their plot. Even more intriguing was that after Oswald shot President Kennedy, he ran from a warehouse (Book Depository) and ran to a theater; Booth, after shooting President Lincoln in a theater ran to a warehouse (barn). It was noted that President Kennedy had a secretary with last name Lincoln and President Lincoln had a secretary whose last name was Kennedy.

President Lincoln is now slumped in his chair and having difficulty breathing. Historians note he was paralyzed at this time and almost everyone else was paralyzed with fear. As fate would have it, Almarin Cooley Richards, Superintendent of the Washington Metropolitan Police was present in the audience the night of the shooting and immediately began investigations. From the back parlor of the house, Richards interviewed witnesses and on the spot and ordered the warrant to arrest Booth.

Several soldiers rushed into the Presidential Box and were instructed to carry Lincoln outside the suite across the street for more privacy and to administer to him better. Among the soldiers carrying President Abraham Lincoln across the street we find a police officer. None other than Joseph Gales and as he clings to the President they make a human stretcher paving their way across the cobblestone street to the adjacent Peterson House. The home is a late Victorian architecture and a 19th Century federal style row house located at 516 10th Street, NW. The house was built in 1849, by a German tailor, Mr. William A. Peterson.

A slight rain began to fall as they carried him and despite chaos all around them one couldn't help but know that God is supreme even in crisis. It is comforting to know when it rains on Earth that He still reign up in Heaven. Joseph Gales and his new friends place the bloodied and battered President on a bed that was too small for his 6'4" frame.

Pillows were placed gingerly but immediately to elevate his head and after what seemed like an eternity the Surgeon General arrived at the house and predicted that the President wouldn't make it through the night. Physicians continued like Lincoln's pocket watch around the clock. They tried relentlessly and removed blood clots that had materialized over the wound and then poured out excess fluid from the brain hoping to relieve pressure. Dr. Anderson Abbott was also one of the attending physicians and he was the first black Canadian granted a medical license.

Mary Todd Lincoln may have seemed aloof at times in their tumultuous marriage but she was now fully engaged this fateful night and she wept so profusely that she had to be escorted out of the bedroom to give both the President and others around him peace of mind. I often wonder if the president could hear anything at this moment and if he did was he comforted that the woman who seemed so distant in life actually cared for him near death?

Vice President Johnson along with members of the Cabinet and a few of Lincoln's closest friends stood and had a prayer vigil. They were faithfully by his side until he breathed his last and was pronounced dead at twenty two minutes after seven in the morning. When the President's heart ceased to beat it was as if time had stood still for America and beyond. Lincoln didn't need a Rolex to remind him that time is short, tomorrow is not guaranteed and a life without urgency equates catastrophe. The President probably had an idea that his life would be cut short and he didn't have time to waste. The Bible talks about "redeeming the time" and Lincoln sure made the most of his while on Earth.

Unbeknownst to Lincoln in an interview published in the New York Times on April 30, 1906 that Doug Stiles, great-great-grandson of watchmaker John Dillon called to corroborate a story that had been passed down for generations in his family. Apparently, Jonathan Dillon was employed for M.W. Galt & Company in 1861 when the owner of the shop announced the first shot of the Civil War had been fired on Fort Sumter. He went on to share the news inspired him to unscrew the dial of President Lincoln's watch which he was repairing at the time and with a sharp tool inscribed on the metal beneath: "The first gun is fired. Slavery is dead." Thank God for a president who will at least try?" And try he did.

The Lord died on Good Friday two thousand years ago to set sinners free; on Good Friday 1865 Abraham Lincoln died after allowing slaves to go free. The end of his time became the beginning for so many and we have much to thank President Lincoln for.

Amidst the tears and heart break President Lincoln's body was placed in a temporary, humble coffin and draped with a flag and escorted by armed cavalry back to the Executive Mansion. Even in death, the president is to be protected. In this case not only protected but respected. The remains of the President, once back at The White House, were exposed and an autopsy was conducted.

Edward Curtis who was employed with U.S. Army as a surgeon recalled hearing a bullet clatter into a basin as the doctor's removed part of Lincoln's brain. He later penned, "The entire medical staff stopped to stare at the offending weapon, "the cause of such mighty changes in the world's history as we may never realize."

Just as the cherry blossom seedlings seemed so small yet blossomed to be such a blessing around the globe; the small, single bullet that Booth used to assassinate Lincoln changed history as well, but for the worse.

The First Lady begged for the surgeon to remove some of his hair as a keepsake. Allegedly, First Lady Jackie Kennedy asked for the same request. Very few doubt the devotion of Jackie to Jack Kennedy but Mary despite depression and demons of her own was more suspect of her devotion to

Honest Abe. Perhaps she wanted to love his locks and feel his hair in death for failing to stroke his hair with appreciation in life.

Even depression subsides in death. Flags were ordered to be flown at half-mast and the entire country mourned the loss of their leader but now no less than 10,000 police and military personnel are looking for the cowardly loser. The world's biggest man hunt is on the prowl for the actor who caused all this drama. Booth had made his way into my hometown of Waldorf, MD (some 28 miles south of the Nation's Capital) and at midnight he and his fellow conspirator, David Herold, knocked on the door of another surgeon by the name of Dr. Samuel Mudd.

Ironically, a great-great-great-grandson of Dr. Mudd and I went to elementary, middle and high school together. Dr. Mudd, took the Hippocratic Oath vowing to assist anybody, anywhere and at any time. Maybe you have heard the expression, "His name is Mudd!" To this day, a century and half later, the late surgeon who assisted John Wilkes Booth in the middle of the night still hasn't had his name exonerated.

The morning after the physician set Booth's broken bone, the men were off and running again. Guilt runs and Lord knows they were wrong. The manhunt intensified and Union troops surrounded a barn on a Virginia farm and soldiers set fire to it hoping to extract the dynamic and deadly duo. As the blaze raged to an inferno, it was Herold who surrendered but Booth was not giving up.

A sergeant shot John Wilkes Booth in the back of the neck because he raised his gun as if to shoot and they carried him out alive. If you live by the sword you often die by it and what goes around comes around. Fitting Oswald died by a gun too. What were the odds just as President Kennedy was taken and pronounced dead at Parkland Memorial Hospital his assassin, Lee Harvey Oswald died in the exact same hospital in the very next emergency treatment room. President Kennedy died in ER One and Oswald in ER Two. What are the odds? The same physician who worked on President Kennedy would also work on Oswald. When you take that oath you are to assist the good, bad and ugly. The doctor didn't want the alleged assassin to be in the same room as the president had died. Therefore, on a moment's notice ushered Oswald to the second emergency room. You probably never thought of this but you can never be first when you live for self. Just ask Satan the loser, Lucifer who tried to be equal with God and was kicked out of Heaven. Pride always goes before the fall.

Booth lasted for three hours before looking at his guilty hands and his dying words were, "Useless, useless!" That statement speaks volumes and personifies powerfully a life poorly lived. Regardless, if selfish because the middle of word sin is "I" and the reward of that behavior is lost, wasted and useless! History reveals and the Bible records the fact that bad guys do not win in the end. The President died with honor and Booth and his buddies died hated by an entire nation. One was famous and the other infamous. We can't forget Lincoln but Booth is not worth remembering. One was a leader and the other died a loser.

President Lincoln was laid in state in the Rotunda of the United States Capitol in Washington, D.C. and eventually placed on a train to his beloved home of Springfield, Illinois. He returned to where it all started. True leaders not only listen but long to go home. Lincoln was no exception.

Do you recall Joseph Gales, the Washington D.C. police officer who had a friendship with President Lincoln and carried him at his death? What you may not know is that his first name was Joseph and his middle name was Gales. His last name was Shelton. Joseph Gales Shelton was my great-great-great-grandfather.

Just as my maternal ancestor hand planted the Cherry Blossoms around the Tidal Basin in 1912, my paternal ancestor almost fifty years before (Good Friday, 1865) hand carried arguably the greatest President we will ever have. One ancestor carried the President and other a plant. Without question, I will go to my grave knowing both when in their presence knew they were with greatness.

My great-grandmother Lillian Lomax lived on 1321 33rd Street in Georgetown between N & 0 during the 1950's and United States Senator John F. Kennedy and Jackie lived on 3307 N Street just half a block away around the corner. My mother, Sharon Lomax as a child would often see young Caroline Kennedy walking with her governess while her father was on Capitol Hill en route to the highest office in the land. Just a couple years later, they moved to The White House.

My father retired as Deputy Chief of the United States Capitol Police and was the senior of the three Deputy Chiefs of the respected department. During his career, he protected six United States Presidents. Dad served on the Inaugural Committee in charge of the security for the swearing in ceremony for President William Jefferson Clinton's first inauguration. January 20, 1993, my mother and I sat in the fifth row as President Clinton was sworn in despite nearly half a million people in attendance on the West Front. At that time, Dad and his colleagues were in charge of providing security for the largest ever inauguration on the West Front. Ironically, the same side of the United States Capitol when Meadowlark and I sat in the chauffeured limousine together.

My Uncle, Lt. Charles Shelton was in charge of the entire K-9 department for the U.S. Capitol Police and for years the K-9 unit has been known to have some of the best dogs and dog handlers in the world. Their father, my grandfather, William Robert Shelton was a Captain with the D.C. Metropolitan Police and for awhile was strategically placed in the balcony of the United States Senate to protect senators while they were in session. My great grandfather, William Franklin Shelton, rode a motorcycle as a police officer with the United States Park Police in DC. My great-great grandfather, Benjamin Franklin Shelton, walked a patrol beat as a D.C. police officer. It was my great-great-great-grandfather, Joseph Gales Shelton who was the first of now five generations of Washington D.C. police officers in our family and they have protected the last twenty six of twenty eight United States Presidents.

Regardless, if working overtime at The White House and befriending Lincoln or assisting with the presidential chariot and now motorcade with bullet proof windows, providing sweeps with bomb sniffing dogs or walking side by side with the leader of the free world, always vigilant and on the lookout, they all in their own way helped provide protection for the President.

When my great-great-great grandfather had the honor to converse with President Lincoln I know he knew he was talking to greatness. When he stood in his presence and looked up to his compassionate yet weary eyes I knew he was cognizant of the fact that he was staring at greatness. When he would be a few steps over the shoulder standing post and providing protection for the most powerful person on the planet I know he was mindful he was securing greatness. The night Lincoln was shot he was one of the first to respond but he was not positioned at the door the night of the assassination. However, when he (Shelton) assisted in carrying him across the street I am certain in that moment during that national storm he knew he was carrying greatness.

With each step in the rain as he and those soldiers tried to comfort him while carrying President Lincoln, I often wonder what went through Shelton's head? Did the training mode kick in and he was trying to secure the scene and get him to a bedroom for safety and surgery? Was he in shock that one of his own friends was injured? Did he recall the long hours alone with the leader of the free world yet divided nation? The jokes that he like all Shelton's practice with precision and pinpoint accuracy with so many other friends and family now recalls the larger than life president after hearing one of his jokes bowing down with laughter that his iconic stove top hat almost fell to the ground?

Did he find solace that for a brief moment he was able to provide a temporal comfort from the war and a wife missing in action that perhaps with his humor and friendship helped Lincoln's days and occasional nights, like his son's name, a "Tad" more bearable? If you don't think the presidency is lonely perhaps some of their own words will clarify. The White House Historical Association record President Gerald Ford saying, "The Executive Mansion is the best public housing I've ever seen." President Harry S. Truman referred to the White House as a "glamorous prison," and the "great white sepulcher of ambitions." Julie Nixon Eisenhower in "Pat Nixon, The Untold Story" shared, "The isolation of the president in the White House is not so much self imposed as it is imposed by others and by the nature of the office itself. The ushers, military aides, and key staff members all try to ensure that the president's energy is reserved for the big decisions; to spare him petty details of life; to fulfill as quickly as possible his requests, large and small. The First Family is similarly isolated and oddly unaware of most of the rumors that sweep through Washington." The Bible reminds us to pray for those in authority because they not only have the same problems as us but often compounded.

Like any selfless servant and protector of the peace, I know that Joseph Gales Shelton while carrying President Abraham Lincoln wished Booth's bullet had hit him instead. To this day, Special Agent Clint Hill who was on the Secret Service detail for President Kennedy fifty years later has relived that moment every day since and would have gladly traded places a million times over.

The irony of ironies is that President Abraham Lincoln established the United States Secret Service on the very day that he was assassinated at Ford's Theater. Its main duty at the time was to prevent illegal production of counterfeit currency. During Lincoln's Administration the monetary process was so disorganized that it was believed that a third of the nation's money was counterfeit. On the recommendation of Treasury Secretary Hugh McCulloch, the President commissioned a task force to stop this problem immediately from further destroying the country's economy.

The Secret Service officially went to work July 5, 1865 (three months after Lincoln's death). The first chief was William Wood who was well respected for his bravery during the Civil War and in that first year helped close more than two hundred counterfeit plants. That success helped prove the value of the Secret Service and in 1866 their national headquarters was established in the adjacent Treasury Building next door to the Executive Mansion. President Lincoln's assassination was the first in our nation but unfortunately not the last. Congress began to re-think and consider adding presidential protection but typical Capitol Hill took an additional thirty-six years and the death of two more U.S. Presidents before they agreed to add protection to the duties of the Secret Service.

Even today too many in society value money more than men and women. Congress allowed agents to stop stolen money but could care less about safeguarding and protecting human beings. The last I checked, mankind is more valuable than money and we all win when we consider others better than ourselves. One hundred and fifty years ago, President Abraham Lincoln had to rely on just a handful of Washington, D.C. policemen working overtime for protection. In 2013, the United States Secret Service now employs over six thousand trained professionals, of which approximately 4,400 are sworn to protect, with an annual budget just shy of two billion dollars.

Just as another scenario danced before this pre-agent's head the slight rain began to pick up and reminded my ancestor while carrying President Lincoln of the task at hand. Either way, when Shelton held President Lincoln in his arms he carried the closest to the king of a nation we will ever have. By George, President Washington was right when he said, "no king but King Jesus!" In 1999, it was my honor to meet the late Helen Thomas, a White House press correspondent who covered every president from John Kennedy to George W. Bush, respectively and I will end this chapter how she concluded each press briefing by saying, "Thank you Mr. President."

My family over the years obtained documents pertaining to my ancestor and these two clippings in Washington, D.C. newspapers reveal some wonderful nuggets in his obituary. The Association for the Preservation of The Historic Congressional Cemetery noted:

"Obituary – Shelton, Joseph G. On Thursday, October 24, 1907 at 2:10 a.m. Joseph G. Shelton in the 79th year of his age. Funeral from his late residence, 406 12th Street, SE on Saturday, October 26 at 2 p.m. Relatives and friends invited.

"The Evening Star, October 25, 1907" – Joseph G. Shelton Dead. Veteran Policeman and Native Washingtonian. Arrangements were completed today for the funeral of Joseph G. Shelton, a veteran policeman, whose death was announced in The Star, yesterday. The interment will be held at Congressional Cemetery. It is said former associates of deceased will act as pallbearers. Joseph G. Shelton resided in Washington since his birth on March 5, 1829 and was identified with nearly every movement for the advancement of the interests in general and East Washington in particular. Appointed a policeman October 18, 1861, soon after the old auxiliary guard had been merged into the first metropolitan police force, he performed the duty of patrolman in the exciting and trying period of the Civil War. He had many thrilling experiences with deserters, bounty jumpers and desperate characters who flocked to Washington during the war period. There was a saying among the police in those days of the fire and smoke of war that there was on any average one murder a day in this city. The policemen were therefore required to perform heroic service.

It is said Mr. Shelton was one of the officers who responded to the call

Patrolman Clements when he arrested single-handed nearly an entire company of Zoeaves were taken to the old central guardhouse on Louisiana Avenue, between 9th and 10th Streets, and there put through "ducking" process. It is explained that the drunken men were placed in small cells and the hose turned on them, deluging them with water until they were sober enough to be released. On the pension roll Mr. Shelton served as a policeman until April 15, 1887 before the era of call boxes and patrol wagons, when owing to physical disability, he was placed on the pension roll of the department. He also retained his membership in the Police Relief Association. He was also stationed at the White House during Civil War, and was frequently detailed as a bodyguard to President Lincoln. His sagacity and bravery won for him high esteem about the city and among the police force where he had many friends. He was on terms of personal friendship with President Lincoln as the result of his position at the Executive Mansion, and was also acquainted with many other famous men of that day. He was stricken with paralysis about three weeks ago without warning while he was conversing with his daughter, Miss Sarah E. Shelton, and fell to the floor. Several times since the attack it was feared he would die, but on each occasion of an apparent relapse he seemed to rally. He gradually lost strength, however, and the end came at ten minutes past 2 o'clock yesterday morning."

The Evening Star, October 2, 1907 - "With Lincoln When He Died." Veteran Policeman Nearing Portal of Death Was at Ford's Theater as Escort When President Was Assassinated. Last night his demise was expected at any moment, and today the attending physicians hold out no hope for his recovery. Mr. Shelton served as an escort and accompanied President Lincoln to Ford's Theater the night he was shot and helped carry the wounded President to the house on the opposite side of the street, where he died. Mr. Shelton is regarded as one of the few remaining landmarks of the old police force nearly half a century ago."

CHAPTER NINE

KING OF ROCK 'N ROLL

After his tenure serving in the United States Army overseas and returning to make films at home his "star" began to rise again. Most professionals are fortunate to have one act but Elvis Presley had multiple stages of success. Early in the 1950's he hit it big and with a string of movies in the early 1960's took him to stardom but like his rank, Private Presley actually feared that his absence in the military may eliminate his fan base upon returning. Truth be told, even the most gifted public artists on stage can still be quite insecure individuals behind the scenes. Elvis later said in an interview, "The image is one thing and the human being is another…. it's very hard to live up to an image."

For any critics who thought Elvis' career was over his recent 1968 "Comeback Special" in his famed black leather suit immediately eliminated those doubts. He had been a star previously but that live performance catapulted him to super stardom and Elvis was back on the map and millions of old and new fans desired and demanded to see him on tour. Elvis missed the instant connection with a live audience. Sure it was nerve wracking but the benefit was unlike any other. In a MGM documentary Elvis in his own words said, "The first time that I appeared on stage, it scared me to death. I really didn't know what all the yelling was about. I didn't realize that my body was moving. It's a natural thing to me. So to the manager backstage I said, 'What'd I do? What'd I do?' And he said "Whatever it is, go back and do it again!"

Elvis mania was sweeping the nation and even the Beatles took a backseat. When he came to town electricity was in the air and people went wild! Very few are known around the globe by their first name (Meadowlark is one and Elvis is another). The "King of Rock & Roll's record sales and sold out concerts are almost second to none. When Elvis and his entire entourage arrived to any city it was nothing shy of a presidential visit equipped with motorcade and all. With Elvis, nothing was small. Elvis Presley in the early 1970's was touring across the United States and one of those stops he was scheduled to perform was in Denver, Colorado

During a sound check a couple hours before the show, Elvis was adorning a black jumpsuit with matching cape on November 17, 1970 and was walking in the corridors of the Denver Coliseum. Desiring to get some rest before the show he jumped in an awaiting limo in the basement of that massive concrete convention center and was rushed up, out and down the road to the Radisson Hotel on 1776 Grant Street. While taking an elevator towards the 10th floor of the hotel he was met by two off-duty Denver police officers employed to provide security for Elvis protection at hotel. Johnny Cash was known as the man in black but now Elvis with jet black hair and matching costume and cape played more the part in that moment.

Similar to President Lincoln and a policeman we find another of America's royalty befriending one. Elvis had a huge heart for and unique interest in law enforcement. He had once said if he hadn't been an entertainer, he would have liked to have been a policeman. Elvis liked to collect honorary badges given to him by local police departments. In fact, President Richard M. Nixon would give Elvis a DEA badge a month later on December 21, 1970 in the Oval Office.

That late afternoon in Colorado, Elvis asked the two policemen if they were going to attend the concert that night. The policeman replied, "I would love to but have to work security behind the scenes for your show." Elvis was never one to take no for an answer, and asked for his supervisor's phone number on the spot and immediately made a call personally not asking for permission but telling the officer's superior that he would have the night off as his personal guest. Elvis didn't get the motto, "TCB" by accident. It meant, taking care of business in a flash and he not only preached it but lived it. The officer was elated and Elvis was one of the few who could pull that off so quickly.

Elvis then looked the police officer square in the eye and asked him did he have any particular favorite song of his? The policeman gave the polite answer that he liked almost all his musical work but said, "How Great Thou Art" was his favorite. Elvis smiled and replied like he always did after almost each song when the crowd approved, "Thank you, thank ya very much." That night the officer who was scheduled to be working off duty at the hotel, thanks to Elvis, he was riding in a limousine en route to the concert with his fellow police partner!

Later that night, Elvis brought the house down and the crowd was beside themselves. In the middle of the concert in front of a capacity crowd Elvis didn't forget his conversation with the cop. From the stage he had the house lights shine on the policeman that he met just a few hours before and as if time stood still he said, "I would like to dedicate this next song to my new friend." My father's friend, Bob Cantwell said later, "Elvis always nailed it on those Gospel songs but I never heard him sing "How Great Thou Art" with such power as he did that night!" For Elvis to sing a hymn in the middle of a rock show took guts, grace and God. Elvis in that moment with the help of the Holy Spirit turned that Colorado concert into a church service with 16,000 other congregants.

The policeman was overwhelmed, the crowd went wild and Elvis as always replied, "Thank ya very much" and moved on to the next song selection like it was no big deal. Looking back, I am uncertain what was more amazing; a cop who had the guts to tell the king of rock n roll to his face that he liked a Gospel song or Elvis at the top of his game actually singing it at his concert in honor of him (Bob) while singing it for Him (Jesus). The greats are gracious and after the show Elvis before leaving town gave Bob a personal autographed picture assuring him he would be in contact. Bob became close friends with him from 1970-1977. So close that Bob continued to work for Elvis and spend personal time with Elvis. They spent several weekends together skiing at Vail, Colorado and Elvis flew him a couple times to Graceland in Memphis, Tennessee.

Elvis despite being known by billions and loved by millions had a gift to make individuals feel loved and respected. He was generous beyond measure and lived to give. Over the years, I have been to both his humble home in Tupelo, Mississippi and the magnificent mansion in Memphis called "Graceland" and what endeared him to so many is he knew all he had was because of God. He recognized that "to whom much was given much is required". Dr. Johnny Hunt is right, "Riches left sitting resemble manure more than money." It "stinks" if we don't share what we have. That will preach!

Bob and Elvis reunited again several months later after that first meeting in Denver but this time "E" paid for him and his wife, Jody to join him in Las Vegas on January 31, 1971. Elvis was playing in concert at the International Hotel and when they arrived personnel escorted Bob and Jody to the front and placed them sitting dead center on the floor next to the stage. When the concert started, the crowd was electric and this time "the king" waltzed on stage wearing his trademark white jumpsuit sporting his slender frame and the women went wild! Once again, Elvis paused in the middle of his show and had the houselights shine on Bob and his wife and then he sang "Sweet Caroline" to his wife and the rest is history. To this day, Jody still remembers that evening. What woman wouldn't?

At that moment, I am not sure who was smiling brighter; the policeman's wife or the man who just recently became a friend for life with a living legend. Having the privilege to grow and know Elvis' step-brother, Rick Stanley, I bet it would be safe to say that Elvis had the greater satisfaction. It was said in a Biblical admonition that "It's better to give than to receive" and you cannot out give God.

My father met Bob at the F.B.I. Academy in Quantico, VA and they graduated together in 1978 (just months after Elvis' death on August 16, 1977.) When Elvis passed, Bob continued his career in law enforcement, and retired as the Deputy Chief of the Denver Police Department. My father retired as Deputy Chief of U.S. Capitol Police. It is a small world and both their faith in God and F.B.I. training helped not hindered the careers of both, respectively. In 1978, Dad brought his new friend home from the Academy one weekend and I was six years old at the time. To put things in perspective, Elvis was HUGE in our house! To have a friend of Elvis Presley under our roof was unbelievable and the icing to my childhood cake. We were so excited to roll out the red carpet that I volunteered that Bob would sleep in my bed and I took the couch. My mentality was "if you are good enough for Graceland than you certainly can stay in my room." I will never forget upon leaving that Bob wrote the kindest hand-written note for forsaking my bed to enable him to rest.

The night before is what I will recall the most. My mom had prepared the best dinner and special dessert and I always wished more guests would come over because she was a good cook but it always got great when visitors were in the house! At six years old my bed time was about

8 PM but that night we stayed in the dining room in Waldorf, Maryland and it seemed like midnight came too quickly as he shared a photo album of his visits to Graceland and story after story of his experiences with Elvis and his friendship with the late rocker.

Honestly, I couldn't get enough and hung on every word. My parents eventually had to pry me to the couch to sleep but even they loved having him visit us. Bob shared about the 1976 Cadillac Seville that Elvis gave him and the countless gifts, guns and jewelry that Presley generously bestowed on not only him, but also on those in his circle and even complete strangers.

Many Elvis fans are familiar with the legendary story of Elvis sitting at Graceland one night and he was known to do things spontaneously and on a dime. When you have money the decisions you make may not always make sense or save cents. Elvis had a craving for a submarine sandwich late one night. The catch is he didn't want one from down the street in Memphis, so Elvis remembered the outstanding sandwich he had eaten while in Denver with his friends on the Denver Police force, including Bob.

Elvis called his police friends in Denver and told him to purchase a six-foot-long peanut butter, bacon and grape sub served on toasted white French bread and get on the next flight to Memphis with it. It was called "Fool's Gold Loaf" and he was introduced to the unique, delicious artery numbing sandwich by Bob and his buddies with the Denver Police Department on a previous visit. Elvis didn't like anyone to tell him no, but Bob told Elvis he was sorry, but there wasn't a commercial airline that would allow him to bring a six foot sub on board. Mom recalls to the best of her recollection that Elvis said some choice words to Bob and hung up.

Elvis called his pilots and told them to get his jet "Lisa Marie" (named after his daughter) ready because he needed to fly to Denver. A few hours later, Lisa Marie landed at Denver Stapleton Airport. Elvis, said to Bob, "You wouldn't bring the sandwich to me, so I came to pick it up myself. The Colorado Mine Company, famous for the Fools Gold sandwich delivered the sandwiches to Elvis at the airport. Elvis said "I'm hungry!" Talk about fast food and I can still hear Elvis saying after eating that meal 33,000 feet in the air, "Thank ya very much."

One night, Elvis couldn't sleep which was par for his course and decided to drive around town. The streets were bare and Elvis came upon a Cadillac dealership and couldn't believe his eyes. He saw an African-American woman alone after midnight staring into the show room dealership on the outside looking in just dreaming "maybe one day."

Elvis parked the car, walked up behind her and politely said in his southern drawl, "Ma'am, do you like that car?" Before even recognizing his voice or turning around to see his face she said, "Indeed I do!" Elvis said to one of the guys behind him, "Get the owner on the phone!" That is all he needed to say because Elvis had frequented there many times and had purchased many cars from the dealership. As usual, Elvis was in the process of taking care of business in a flash one more time. Previously when meeting Bob in Colorado he called his supervisor immediately now back home in Tennessee he is calling the car dealership owner. Most businessmen would be irate or offended if awakened from sleep in the middle of the night but when Elvis called it was not only fun but meant commission sales!

When Elvis called everyone said, "Thank ya very much!" Elvis had bought dozens of Cadillac cars for family, friends and again in this case for a complete stranger. The owner arrived and they wheeled that Cadillac off the showroom floor and Elvis handed her the keys with a smile. Her "one day" was that morning just minutes past midnight and once again, despite her beaming ear to ear it, was Elvis who had the bigger smile because it really is better to give than to receive.

If he heard of someone that needed money for utility bills, he not only paid that month's bill but would pay nearly the next year in advance. If they needed surgery, he was known to pick up the bill personally and get square with the hospital. When one of his back-up singers learned while on tour with Elvis that his colleague's home was burglarized, Elvis caught the next flight home with his employee beside him and personally consoled the wife, told the kids that he would make it up to them and replaced everything brand new. Looking back, it was a blessing because what was old became new when Elvis followed through.

One of the Stamps Quartet singers said one night on tour the crew grew nervous because right before the show started Elvis was nowhere to be found. The staff and security looked high and low and couldn't find "The Big E." Panic set in and the "2001" Theme song had already started blaring with nearly 18,000 ecstatic fans and Elvis is missing in action!

Someone looked into a janitor's closet and what they found was none other than Elvis Presley on his hands and knees in jumpsuit, scarf and cape begging God as if he were a preacher to give him power from above to minister to the crowd out front. It was as if he knew two things -- Elvis had a gift from God and without Heavenly intervention he personally would have nothing to give the awaiting crowd.

Perhaps the story that touched me the most was despite having two personal jets, Elvis on rare occasion would fly on a commercial flight like anyone else. One particular night they were coming back from a West Coast trip on the now defunct Trans World Airlines (TWA) and Elvis and his entourage was sitting in First Class. It was a red eye flight home to Memphis and a stewardess hesitantly came up to Elvis and said: "Sir, we have a problem. The word has gotten out that you are on this flight. We cannot land because the coach class is going crazy. Will you kindly come through the curtain and say hello to the passengers?"

Elvis responded with a smile and knowing his services were needed didn't see it as an inconvenience but another assignment and said, "Sure." Elvis unbuckled his seatbelt, walked through the curtain separating first class from coach and "the king" held court 33,000 feet above the ground. Just like he did at Madison Square Garden, or at the car dealership, he now held this captive audience on the airplane in the palm of his hand. He rested his arm on the back of a seat while waving to the crowd and forgot that he was wearing a ring on every finger. He recently heard that Liberace bought a massive ring and not to be outdone Elvis bought one larger. All of his rings were nice but this one in particular was so large it resembled a Super Bowl ring. It literally took up two fingers and was filled with massive diamonds.

As his right hand dangled in front of this particular row conversing with the crowd equipped with a middle age, attractive woman she was looking at Elvis. Her seven-year- old son was not looking at his face but rather at his fingers and couldn't get his eyes off the "bling" that "the king" (Elvis) was wearing. At this juncture, Elvis probably forgot he was wearing all those diamonds but then again he didn't ask to speak to this capacity crowd on a commercial jet. Since he was the consummate southern gentleman he couldn't turn it down the opportunity or being poverty stricken as a youth like his song "couldn't let the poor boy down."

Elvis was turning to exit after saying "goodnight" and the little boy grabbed him by the satin shirt and said, "Sir, you must be someone really important." Elvis stood still and said, "Son, why do you say that?" The child replied, "I don't know who you are or what you do but you must have a pretty good job." Elvis, really shocked by his statement said, "What do you mean?" The lad replied with a child like faith, "I sure hope I can get a job like you someday so I can buy a ring like the one you are wearing." Elvis didn't hesitate and asked, "What ring are you talking about?" The boy said, "Mister, all of them are nice but that one right there is H-U-G-E!" The child was pointing to the one that took up two fingers and said, "Sir, that's the one I would like to buy!!" Once again, Elvis smiled and said with the entire plane watching: "Son, you won't have to and this is my gift to you." He took off the massive diamond ring and laid it on the boy's fold-down tray and walked back to the first class section of the plane and like at every sold out concert the curtain closed behind him.

The passengers in coach class were left speechless and the boy went bonkers as Elvis sat down like it was no big deal. When Elvis dedicated "How Great Thou Art" to Bob in Colorado it was no big deal to him. When he gave the Cadillac to the woman at midnight in Memphis to him it was no big deal and just giving a ring worth tens of thousands of dollars to a young boy while flying somewhere over the middle of the country it was no big deal to Elvis. One of the bodyguards sitting next to Elvis leaned over and whispered "E!" Some of us have been willing to take a bullet for you for a couple years. Why didn't you give us the ring?" Elvis replied, "Man, you never asked!" As always, he gave and helped others until it hurt him.

The National Archives note that the most famous photograph in their possession is the one taken of Elvis on the day he went to The White House for a meeting with President Richard M. Nixon. Elvis on the spur of the moment again was not one to sit idle and when he had an idea he had to "take care of business." He wanted to go under the radar but it is next to impossible when you are arguably the most recognized face in the world. If you haven't learned by now, if Elvis wanted something or someone, he made it happen in a flash.

The truth is even though Elvis was very wealthy, he didn't always carry a credit card nor had a clue how to manage the basic necessities in life. He had people employed to do those things but because he had to leave immediately he showed up unannounced at Memphis International Airport dressed to the nines. People starred with their mouths dropped in awe and couldn't believe their native son was flying on a normal plane like everyone else. When he approached the ticket counter the woman almost fainted as her heart pounded to see the handsome hunk right before her very eyes.

Good thing she didn't die because he needed her assistance immediately and he had a plane to catch but didn't book his flight in advance. To make matters more complicated, he not only was without a credit card but also without his identification. Fortunately, his fame could be a blessing and a burden but this time it worked in his favor and she happily let him on the plane because everyone knew who he was! The funny thing was he didn't even know how the credit card worked he just hoped the transaction would go through not because of a lack of funds but he rarely got out alone without ten men handling his transactions.

With no time to spare, Elvis boarded a non-stop flight to the Nation's Capital and with no hotel reservations he went "by faith." My mother always said: "God looks after children, good people and dummies" and at times I have been all three. Elvis had the time of his life without his entourage and was a kid in the candy store! People stared at him the entire flight and seeing him then at National Airport caused more of a stir now than a hundred Elvis impersonators in Vegas. Folks expect it now but when you are the original people are not expecting to see you out and about.

Elvis checked into "Hotel Washington" and exactly two decades later my prom date and I had dinner on the top floor of that same famous landmark. It is less than two blocks away from The White House and Elvis wrote a handwritten note on his stationary and sent it to the Secret Service informing them that he was in town and requested a meeting with the President.

If you have ever tried to get a meeting with the most powerful person in the world, let's just say it is not the easiest date to get on a calendar. Once again, Elvis didn't know any different and Presley wasn't worried about Presidential protocol. Ironically half of America viewed him "the king" with more clout than the current president. While things would prove difficult or even impossible for the average Joe, everything tended to fall into place for Elvis. Sure enough, he received word that President Nixon would meet him the next day!

Elvis left Memphis so quickly that he didn't even bring a change of clothes but when you got to go – you gotta go! Elvis was gone and now en route the next day to 1600 Pennsylvania Avenue. By this time two of his dear friends caught planes and Jerry Schilling, his long time aide and assistant flew in from Los Angeles on a "red eye" and was there in Washington to accompany Elvis the day "the king met the President."

Even the Secret Service agents were huge fans of Elvis when he walked through the gates and his bodyguards didn't want to relinquish the revolvers that they were carrying. Elvis came prepared with ammunition but not clothes; but in his eyes he had his priorities straight. Elvis is adorning a purple velvet suit with matching cape and sporting a Napoleon white high collar that was custom made just for him. Plus, he was wearing rings fit for royalty and wearing the 24kt solid gold belt that he was awarded in Las Vegas for breaking the all-time sell out record.

An aide escorted Elvis and his friends to the West Wing and the next thing they know is the thick door opens and they are now stepping inside the Oval Office. Elvis had a jungle room in Tennessee and President Nixon had his own in Washington. Elvis dressed to kill (while reluctantly leaving his guns behind) waltzed in because he rarely walked and now the poor boy from Tupelo is toe to toe with the President of the United States of America. After small talk the conservative President with Quaker roots sized Elvis up and down and trying to be respectful looked at the rock star that resembled "Batman" with the purple cape and said, "Elvis, that's quite an outfit you've got there." Without missing a beat, Elvis smiled and said in his awe shucks style, "Mr. President, you got your show and I got mine."

What Elvis was trying to imply was he knew he had greatness deposited in him and was being authentic to who he was and was respectful of how President Richard Nixon rolled. Only Elvis could get away with what he did and it was at that meeting that President Nixon arranged for Elvis to receive the honorary D.E.A. badge that he desperately desired.

Just a year or two later, my godmother Judy Henderson who led my mother to the Lord when I was an infant had a profound impact on our early walk with Christ. She could be considered a chaplain to the rich and famous. She took me to Hollywood, CA to meet Sylvester Stallone in 1985 when I was thirteen years old and together we presented him a Bible and a drawing that I drew with the plan of salvation on the back. A decade before that meeting with Sly she waited for an entire day in the hotel lobby of a fancy hotel in Los Angeles and gave Elvis a Bible personally. He was looking more handsome than ever with a recent Hollywood tan, chiseled jaw and jet black hair wearing his trademark high collar adorning gold Aviator sunglasses. Elvis said to Judy after receiving the Bible, "Thank you honey. Thank ya very much" and the king kissed her on the cheek.

On another occasion, Elvis was playing a concert at Notre Dame University and an entire row of college students stood up simultaneously with a sign that said, "Elvis, you're The King!" In the middle of the show, he immediately stopped on a dime and pointed to the college kids,

"I am not the King, Jesus Christ is The King!" They sheepishly sat down and he continued the concert. Elvis certainly was human and had his shortcomings like everyone but deep inside I am convinced he knew that he was entrusted with a God given gift and he was carrying greatness within.

One of the reasons that Elvis gave away countless scarves to his fans is because he wanted to touch them and allow them to have a piece of him. When he gave away a scarf he gave part of himself and he hoped it would somehow inspire them to chase their dreams and leave them better than he found them.

In the darkest days of his life, Elvis knew that it was the Lord who carried him. One of his favorite songs was the gospel classic penned by Bill Gaither entitled, "He Touched Me." At night when the crowds went home, Elvis would summon his back-up singers and all he wanted to do to unwind was sing Gospel. They often sang early into the next morning and he never got a Grammy for rock or blues but he won three for his Gospel recordings.

My parents took me twice in 1977 to see Elvis in concert. One was at the Capital Centre in Landover, Maryland and other was Baltimore Convention Center weeks before his death. At one concert Dad had great tickets about ten rows from the floor and on occasion Elvis would pause and invite fans to come towards the stage. My parents had me dressed up in an Elvis jumpsuit that Mom made and Dad escorted me towards the stage. At five years old, in the middle of my childhood hero's concert my father tried to put me right near Elvis hoping he would hoist me up on stage. In front of 17,000 screaming fans, Elvis was reaching right for me at the Capital Centre but he grabbed the child directly next to me. Some have speculated that he picked up a relative of the owner of the arena. So close but so far away! We were feet away from Elvis! Even as kid, I frequently gave concerts to all my friends and I flipped my toy box upside down to become my stage and a Lincoln Log was my makeshift microphone. After my parent's softball games and bowling outings they would often bring friends to the house and in middle of their miniature party I would crank out Elvis records and asked to give a concert. Folks loved it and to this day if Elvis would have picked me up on stage with my costume and handed me the microphone this ham would have done "Hound Dog" and sent that stadium to the moon! Every crowd loves a kid!! If I may quote

Elvis, "Thank ya very much!"

One of his step-brothers had one of the last full conversations before Elvis died in August of 1977. While in his bedroom the stepbrother asked Elvis, "I got a problem. My girlfriend tells me non-stop I need Jesus as my Lord and Savior. What do you think of that?" Elvis often thought his generous acts were "no big deal" but when it came to God or salvation it was important. Perhaps that is why he was offended when playing at Notre Dame others implied he was God. Elvis looked at his stepbrother square in the eye and said, "She is absolutely right. Anyone that has the guts to tell you about Jesus is someone who really cares for you and you need to listen to what she is saying."

Within a day, Elvis was dead. When Elvis passed at the age of 42, he left a fan base around the world in total shock and utterly devastated. Folks passed out from grief, others wanted to die and some wondered if life would ever be the same. The man who was known around the globe by billions and admired by millions, died alone in the bathroom. It is a huge honor to be asked to be a pallbearer at a funeral and it means that of all the people they knew one must have been pretty close to have been asked to carry their casket to the grave.

Dad's friend, Bob was asked to be an honorary pallbearer at Elvis Presley's funeral. The policemen whom Elvis met in Colorado prior to his concert and now having spent seven years with him off and on prior to his death was asked by Vernon Presley (Elvis father) to fly to Memphis and participate in the funeral. Vernon asked Bob to stand guard at the foot of the casket during the funeral service inside Graceland. Just as Secret Service protected presidents in life and death, Bob from Denver is now assigned to protect and respect Elvis in life and his death. What an honor.

That afternoon, approximately seventeen white Cadillac were on hand for the motorcade towards the cemetery and Mr. Presley placed Dad's friend, Bob and a couple of his police friends one of the limos close to the hearse. As the "Memphis Mafia" members carried the remains of his friend who happened to be the late "King of Rock n Roll."

As the world watched and helicopters filmed aerial views, it was as if the President of the United States of America had died. The man who dazzled the world with his voice, captivated crowds by his charisma and lavished his generosity to so many was the poor boy from Tupelo who lived the elusive American Dream. Elvis touched Bob in life and Bob was touching his casket as others carried him in death. Like both Presidents Lincoln and Kennedy, Presley was gone way too soon. Initially, I considered titling this chapter from Yul Brenner's "The King & I" while sharing accounts of our family friend's relationship with Elvis Presley.

Eventually Elvis' remains were removed to Graceland for security purposes so folks wouldn't try to dig up his grave and also so that his body would be located next to his mother, Gladys who was buried at Graceland. He was close to his Momma in life and fitting to be reunited in death; not only in Heaven but on Earth.

Today, over half a million people visit 3734 Elvis Presley Boulevard annually, and enter the gates of Graceland. More tourists visit his house than any other in the world second to only the White House. For the millions who considered Elvis as American royalty are not wrong after all. Most are unfamiliar with these facts that Elvis Presley was a distant cousin of President Jimmy Carter and a direct descendant of Abraham Lincoln's great-great grandfather, Isaiah Harrison. Immediately following Elvis death, President Jimmy Carter said, "Elvis Presley's death deprives our country of a part of itself. He was unique, irreplaceable. More than twenty years ago, he burst upon the scene with an impact that was unprecedented and will probably never be equaled. His music and his personality, fusing the styles of white country and black rhythm and blues, permanently changed the face of American popular culture. His following was immense. And he was a symbol to people the world over of the vitality, rebelliousness and good humor of this country."

The epitaph that Vernon Presley, Elvis' father, wrote on his son's tombstone behind his Memphis mansion sum it up best: "ELVIS AARON PRESLEY - He had a God given gift that he shared with the world. God saw that he was tired and called him Home." Ironically, Elvis on his last tour left the stage with these words, "Till we meet again, may God bless you. Adios." Thanks for the memories and we all can say to Elvis, "Thank you, thank ya very much."

CHAPTER TEN

KING OF ALL KINGS

Black Friday is not the day after Thanksgiving when millions go shopping at an ungodly hour. The original Black Friday was when the God of the universe was crucified at Calvary two thousand years ago on another Friday and the whole world turned dark when The Light was temporarily extinguished.

The temple veil had just ripped and most of His male disciples had already split. The wind blew, the ground shook and the soldiers took what they could. The irony is the guards had just gambled for the garments of God. Appropriate that they gambled for them because religion implies you come to God by buying, earning, laboring or winning but salvation in Christ is free! We are saved by faith and grace not labors or lottery. Sadly, the soldiers knew His clothes were worth something but didn't ponder that His crucifixion and future resurrection granting salvation meant anything. They were so close yet so far away.

While the men were missing in action the women who assembled at the foot of the cross did two things, both starting with "w." They were weeping and worshipping their Lord. Perhaps they were the very first Women of Faith. Sheila Walsh would like that!

It began to rain and some suggest that it was tears from Heaven when God died. One part of the Trinity was gone and the rest wept. The Bible says, "God couldn't look at sin" and perhaps the reason for the darkness that covered the Earth is when God the Father in Heaven turned His back on His only Son at the cross. That moment, despite broad daylight the sun ceased shining and the Savior of mankind died. However, even in death the Son of God never shone brighter. Fallen humanity taught Him how to die but He taught us how to live. I am convinced that when Mary birthed Jesus the moment Christ crawled from out of the crib He was already crawling to our cross.

For those who think that Jesus is either weak or a wimp know neither Christ nor are they a true Christian. God is no weakling but a Warrior! When you are The Way you don't look for an escape route. Jesus led, bled and for three days was dead that we could graduate from a religion in our head to a relationship in our hearts with Almighty God. Even when it rains, Jesus still reigns! Jesus was not some delusional Dictator, nor a misguided Messiah or just a poetic Prophet. Josh McDowell was right when he said, "He is either, Liar, Lunatic or Lord" but you cannot be all of them!

Jesus was not just a teacher or preacher but a reacher rescuing and redeeming lost humanity to His Father. Christ alone is Divinity. He was more than good but Jesus alone is God. The American Dream is graduating from rags to riches but Jesus left riches to rags. He who was worshipped above would be rejected below. He was fully Deity but birthed miraculously of a virgin to be part of humanity. He had a Heavenly Father and earthly mother and left a mansion in Heaven to be born in a manger on Earth. A native of Beulah Land but birthed again in Bethlehem removing His Royal Robes for our ripped rags and at times had no place to lay His head. He vacated the throne to adorn a crown of thorns and the One who poured a zillion gallons of water in the sea thirsted on the cross at Calvary. The Bread of Life who fed thousands hungered alone in the wilderness.

Elvis could relate to living the American Dream. He wore a sequined cape but Jesus was accustomed to a splintered cross. Elvis gave away scarves but Christ with scars gave away eternal life. The greatest entertainer known to man was correct to say there is "only one King." He got it right but Satan got it wrong. It is blasphemy and the height of arrogance for the created to think they are superior to the Creator.

The night that President Lincoln died as my ancestor carried him across the street a light rain fell covering the Washington cobblestone. As the winds subsided and the rain stopped while most men were fearing for their lives behind closed doors a brother from another mother walked up to Pontius Pilate and begged for the Body of his Lord. God gave grace and Joseph of Arimathea had guts. Will the real men and women stand up because the days of sitting down are over and out the window!

Joseph stared Pilate eye to eye and without blinking demanded the body of Christ. Ironically, God used a virgin womb with Mary and a virgin tomb of Joseph of Arimathea to be the "bookends" of the Gospel. Joseph and a few friends then carried Christ from Golgotha to the Garden Tomb.

The distance from the Place of a Skull where Christ was crucified and the Garden Tomb is the length of a football field. Over the years, I often wonder what went through the mind of Joseph of Arimathea at this moment. What was Jesus' step-father thinking at this moment? In the second chapter of this book I gave you a Cup of Joe but we find another Joseph and now serve you a Bowl of Joe who was bold enough to ask for the now deceased Christ.

As Joseph and his makeshift pallbearers carry Christ walking away from Pilate I am curious. Did he think he made a mistake? Did he have faith to start but now feared he should quit thinking Pilate and his police force may now follow and kill them all as they walk away with their God? At any second, did his own safety not even come to question when he saw firsthand the beaten, battered and bloodied body of the One who made time and ironically, now of His own choosing no longer lived. Lincoln had a pocket watch but the Lord didn't need one to remind Him that his days were numbered. His time had come and He was born for this moment.

The Bible says, "No one took His life but He laid it down voluntarily" and if we learn anything from history you cannot keep a good man down much less the God Man. Thugs couldn't keep Joseph down because of his coat and certainly not Jesus because of a cross. Evil never comes in first place in the grand scheme of things. We learn those lessons with the assassin Oswald who was in room number two of that Dallas hospital. Losers will always be last and sinners always second when it is all said and done. Some may have their day in the sun but will have to testify and be judged by the soon returning Son. Those who don't meet Jesus as the Lamb will stand before Him as the

Lion of the Tribe of Judah.

Perhaps Joseph with each step as he carried Christ visualized Jesus asleep in a boat, hoisting children over His Head with a smile wider than the Gaza Strip. Yes the shortest verse in Scripture is, "Jesus wept." Yes, Christ cried but the Savior often smiled and Lord knew laughter too! Maybe He recalled the compassion of Christ as He touched the lepers, befriended the lonely and recruited rejects like Zacchaeus and so many others who were far from Heaven but now found hope and eternal acceptance because of Him. Joseph probably recalled the recent news story of the woman caught in adultery and yet the Just Judge (Jesus) didn't condemn but pardoned her. Admirably and gracefully, Jesus, the Rock of Ages, never threw a rock, the Prince of Peace never tossed a pebble and the Savior, now dead in his arms, never slung a stone. That is not only good but God.

With each step on the dusty, dirty hill country walking towards that vacant tomb the weight of the Lord much less the moment in history began to get heavy. I have always said, "Living up to history can be heavy but missing your Divine destiny is deadly." At this juncture, we see Joseph and his helpers are fatigued trying to carry the crucified Christ and like my ancestor planting the cherry blossoms were probably tempted to slow down, rest or worse even quit. While some doubted the worth of a gift from Japan, these dedicated men couldn't deny and knew that Jesus was worth everything!

As they pondered all that Christ had done for them did they think for a second to give anything less than their best? The song "He's Not Heavy He's My Brother" was a modern day classic but before records were recorded did the thought "He's not heavy, He's my Savior" come to mind as they carried forward? The "Footprints" poem reminds us in the darkest days of our lives it is tempting to see only one set of prints and we ask ourselves, "Where is God in all of this?" The fact is it is in those moments that He is actually carrying us.

As Joseph and his associates carried Jesus in the New Testament I am reminded of another Joseph in the Old Testament despite a band of brothers that were more enemies than family. What propelled him to go on? Why didn't he quit when it was easier to do so? Why keep going when it seems the odds are against you, the stakes are high and the crowd is no longer cheering for your success but demise? I am convinced that both of them knew they were carrying greatness. Joseph, the husband to Mary also had to honor their relationship by faith because as she carried Christ in her womb and ultimately taught him how to clean His room he had to trust that together they were molding, shaping and entrusted to carry greatness.

When David practiced in private and became a warrior in the wilderness with his slingshot he had to realize that he possessed a great gift with an accuracy that was both anointed and appointed for a time such as this. Perhaps all these Gospel giants danced in their heads as they carried Christ from the cross to His temporal tomb.

God now despite dead was Divinity but Joseph was very much human and probably short of breath. As they tried to get a better grip on God wrapping their hands around a body that was raw meat and oozing with blood and bodily fluid found it hard to get a good hold of Him. However, as they held Him they were holding Heaven and Heaven held them. Fortunately, God had a hold of them and they couldn't drop Him because no one could pluck them out of His righteous, right Hand. These were men on a mission and as they carried the Messiah towards the tomb, I will go to my grave convinced that they knew to the core of their very being that they were carrying greatness. It was not an afterthought but at the forefront of their minds. With each step, they were not only part of history but His Story. Mary may have been the first on Earth to carry the Gospel but Joseph of Arimathea and his friends towards that tomb would not be the last. When they carried the Gospel they actually carried God. Ironically, when we carry the Gospel we find God carries us. The movie, "The Godfather" to millions is a cinema classic. If you recall the puppet strings on the poster it implied the hands of the Godfather behind the scenes who called the shots. I submit to you that the nailed scarred Father in Heaven is not behind the scenes but very much on the scene not only calling the shots but carrying us when we cannot carry on.

Two centuries later we learn of a radical remnant called the Pony Riders' Express. They were officially the original mail carriers and were a unique group. The fact is they often rode alone by horseback, harassed by Indians, chased by Cowboys and had to weather the harsh heat in summer and bone chilling cold in winter. They lacked fellowship, were exposed to extreme conditions and their pay was not prosperous.

It was rare that one could catch up with them because, like eagles, they often soared alone. It wasn't that they were arrogant or aloof but their job kept them going nonstop individually. A reporter was able to slowly connect with them one at a time and unbeknownst to the other riders asked them each individually the exact same questions. To the reporter's surprise, he got the same answers. The reporter inquired, "Why do you leave family who love you to reach out to folks who don't know you? Why leave the comfort of your own home for an unpredictable and unsafe life? Why endure hostility and harm when you can relax at your house with no threats? Why face uncertain weather and be gone for extended periods of time regionally, nationally and even globally opposed to maximizing your life locally like everyone else? With tears in each of the Pony riders' eyes they all said one by one to the reporter, "the reason is because the message (mail) we have been entrusted to carry is worth it all." No doubt, many in ministry (especially evangelists) can relate to those Pony Express riders.

To think that Joseph of Arimathea literally had a hand in carrying greatness and the Gospel is the highest high known to man. One doesn't need crack cocaine when you have Christ. A true high is being linked to the Most High God and LSD has nothing on the Lord. For as long as I can remember hearing these stories from my parents and relatives at reunions as a child even today I often think of my ancestors. One carried the Commander- in- Chief (Lincoln) and other planted and protected a plant (cherry blossoms). That night in the light rain on Good Friday, 1865 my paternal ancestor carrying the nearly life-less President and my maternal ancestor nearly half a century later trying to bring life to seedlings that seemed so small. Without question, the answer is I believe both knew they were carrying greatness in the process.

If my ancestor, Joseph Gales Shelton was alive today he would say that it is one thing to carry greatness but entirely and eternally different when greatness carries you. When he carried President Abraham Lincoln he held the closest to a king of a nation America will ever have. The Presidency is an institution not an individual. In August 1977, when our family friend, Bob was a sentry at Elvis casket and named an honorary pallbearer with a select group of men carrying the remains of Elvis Presley, they carried the king of rock 'n roll but Joseph of Arimathea and a few others carried the King of all kings! Today, those that profess Christ as Lord and Savior carry Him daily by their life and lips but because He is alive today; it is Jesus that carries us!

I remember something Dr. Clyde Box said twenty years ago when I sat in the pastors' conference in North Carolina where I was driving Dr. Lee Roberson to the meetings. One of the modern day Prince of preachers said,

"Scholars and skeptics have debated for years if Jesus were simply a man or was He God? He is both! If He wasn't a man then who was that Babe born in Bethlehem? But if He wasn't God, why did thousands of angels sing at his birth? If He wasn't a man, who was that who cried on Calvary's cross, 'I thirst!' But if He wasn't God, why did He tell the woman at the well, 'If you drink from Me you will never thirst again!' If He wasn't a man then who was that dead for three days in Joseph of Arimathea's tomb? But if He wasn't God, explain to me why that tomb is empty?"

Those words are timeless and ring true today. Dr. Box preached one of the greatest sermons I have ever heard "The Napkin." He says he found it in a very old book in his personal library. Most Jewish historians don't debate it but some scholars have some issues but the content is powerful. Excerpts of Dr. Box sermon are found in stores, online, YouTube but this was found on Grace Baptist Church in Decatur, IL on their website.

"In Bible days, when someone died, it was the duty of a family member to close the eyes and kiss the cheek of the dead. When Christ died, this became the duty of two men: Joseph of Arimathea, and Nicodemus. They went to Pontius Pilate and begged the body of the Lord Jesus. Then they had to take Him down from the cross…which was not an easy chore. First, they had to rig a ladder, and climb up the side of the cross, and then they had to pull His hands off over the nails. There was no way they could get those spikes out of the wood, not from that angle, not w/ His hands in between the wood and the nail head. Once the hands were loosed,

they allowed the body of Jesus to sag into a sheet, and would then remove His feet from the nail in the same manner.

They took the body of Jesus to a new tomb that Joseph had prepared for himself. They washed His body, and wrapped it in white linen, folding His arms over His chest. They closed His eyes, kissed His cheek, and placed a napkin over His face. They walked away from that tomb, and no doubt they walked in silence...so that all you could hear was the sounds of their sadness muffled crying, and sniffing. Surely it must have felt like a huge ball of lead in the pit of their stomachs, as they were thinking, "it's all over, the end of the dream...and it only lasted for three short years. Three days passed like an eternity...and I believe with all my heart that the birds refused to sing, and the sun refused to shine. For three days, all the demons of hell rejoiced, and Satan and the forces of darkness thought they had won a great victory. For three days, the Jewish leaders, as well as the Roman government, congratulated themselves on their brilliant scheme. But on the third day, something wonderful and miraculous happened, as God the Father said to an angel in heaven, "Go get Him!" And when the angel's feet hit the ground, the stone rolled away, and up from the grave He arose...He lives!

In our text, Mary comes first to the empty tomb. She sees the stone rolled away and it frightens her. And so she runs to get Peter and John, and they run together to the tomb as fast as they could. John outran Peter, and when he got there, he looked inside, and saw those grave clothes lying there in disarray. Then Peter arrived and, just as we'd expect of him, went right in. He also saw the linen clothes lying there, but there was something unusual in that scene. Something caught their eye that was very interesting. The Gospel of John tells us that the napkin, which was placed over the face of Jesus, was not just thrown aside like the grave clothes. The Bible takes an entire verse to tell us that the napkin was neatly folded, and was placed at the head of that stony coffin. Is that important? You'd better believe it! Is that significant? Absolutely! Is it really significant? Yes!

In order to understand the significance of the folded napkin, you have to understand a little bit about Hebrew tradition of that day. The folded napkin had to do with the Master and Servant, and every Jewish boy knew this tradition.

When the servant set the dinner table for the master, he made sure that it was exactly the way the master wanted it. The table was furnished perfectly, and then the servant would wait, just out of sight, until the master had finished eating, and the servant would not dare touch that table, until the master was finished.

Now if the master were done eating, he would rise from the table, wipe his fingers, his mouth, and clean his beard, and would wad up that napkin and toss it onto the table. The servant would then know to clear the table. For in those days, the wadded napkin meant, "I'm done". But if the master got up from the table, and folded his napkin, and laid it aside his plate, the servant would not dare touch the table, because the servant knew that the folded napkin meant, "I'm not finished yet." The folded napkin meant, "I'm coming back!" Excuse me while I shout (Baptist style). Peter and John had walked with Christ for three years. They had watched as He opened blind eyes and deaf ears. They watched as He literally raised people from the dead. Then they watched Him die…and as they watched, all of their hopes, all of their dreams were shattered! All they could think was, "It's over, it's all over!" And for three long days they were in the depths of despair…the lights of their soul had gone dim. Peter even said," I'm goin' fishin'. I'm going back to what I used to do.

Then after three days, they saw an empty tomb. Not only did they see an empty tomb, but they saw a folded napkin in that empty tomb! I believe with all my heart that when they saw that folded napkin God spoke to them in their being and said, "He's not finished yet…He's coming back!"

I thank God today that He's not finished yet! The tomb is empty, our Savior is alive and the napkin is still folded! I submit to you today that God is not finished saving souls! The folded napkin says that He's not finished saving souls. The Bible says that Jesus came into this world for one reason: to save sinners. John 3:17, "For God sent not his Son into the world to condemn the world; but that the world through him might be saved." Acts 4:12, "Neither is there salvation in any other: for there is none other name under heaven given among men, whereby we must be saved." For that reason, there are two kinds of people in alive today. And the distinction is not black and white…for God doesn't see us that way regardless if we are rich or poor, educated or uneducated and not Republican or Democrat. In the eyes of God, there are two and only two kinds of people: Those that have already been saved and those who need to be saved.

Many people have the mistaken idea that good people ARE saved and only bad people NEED to be saved. Certainly bad people NEED to be saved…and so do "good" people! May I say as clearly as possible, that no one exists who's so bad they CAN'T be saved…and no one so good they don't NEED to be saved! Romans 3:23: "For all have sinned, and come short of the glory of God." In God's eyes, there's no difference…there are no big sinners and little sinners, just sinners. In God's eyes, I'm as guilty of breaking God's holy standard as is Osama bin Laden. In God's eyes, there are sinners who have been forgiven…like me, and sinners who have not been…but certainly CAN be.

Years ago, the great evangelist Billy Sunday was preparing to go into a certain city to do a major crusade. He wrote ahead of time to the mayor of the city, and said, "Would you please send me the names of people in your area who need serious spiritual help". To Sunday's surprise, the mayor sent him…the telephone book! That mayor knew something. He understood that we all need spiritual help. The napkin is still folded…He's still saving souls! Secondly, because the napkin is still folded…He's not finished reclaiming backsliders! A few days before Christ died, He took His disciples aside and told them what was about to happen. He said, I'm going to be betrayed, arrested, beaten, and crucified. Then he looked at the disciples and said, all of you are going to desert me when the heat is on.

The Apostle Peter rose up in typical style and said, Not me, Lord. "Though all shall be offended, yet will I never be offended." In other words, Lord, I don't know about the rest of these bums, but you can count on me! Then he said, "Though I should die with thee, yet will I not deny thee." Can't you just see Jesus shaking his head, saying, "Peter you're going to deny me three times by morning!" Then the Roman soldiers came to arrest the Lord Jesus…with swords, shields and spears. And courage welled up in Peter's heart, and he took out his sword, and even took a swing at them. He lopped off the ear of one of them…and I doubt he was aiming for his ear! The Lord did something incredible. He said, friends, Romans, countrymen, lend me your…no that's a different book!

Seriously, he picked up that ear, and supernaturally reattached it to the man's head. I don't know about you, but if I was a Roman soldier that day, and I saw that miracle, I would have changed sides! "Hey fellas, I came with you, but

I'm leaving with Him!" They arrested Jesus and subjected Him to shear torture. And while this was happening, Peter's courage turned to butter. A young lady approached and said, "I know you, you were with Him". And this same man who had just stood up to the entire Roman army, now backed down and said, "I don't know the man!" Another came up and said the same, and again he denied Christ. Yet another said, your accent betrays you, you're a Galilean, you're one of His disciples, and he not only denied Christ that third time, but for emphasis threw in a few cuss words…I don't know the blankety-blank man, leave me alone! And the rooster immediately crowed, and Peter remembered the words of Jesus. And he looked off into the distance, and there stood Christ, and their eyes caught. And when he saw the sadness and sorrow in the eyes of Jesus, it broke His heart.

He went out to a rock and pounded on it and said, "Oh God, how could I have done this…how can you ever forgive me?" And for three days he lived in shame, guilt, and misery, realizing he had denied the Lord.

Listen now let me drop a blessing in your heart. Look at Mark's account of the Easter story, in Mark 16:1-7: "And when the Sabbath was past, Mary Magdalene, and Mary the mother of James, and Salome, had bought sweet spices, that they might come and anoint Him. And very early in the morning the first day of the week, they came unto the sepulchre at the rising of the sun. And they said among themselves, Who shall roll us away the stone from the door of the tomb? And when they looked, they saw that the stone was rolled away: for it was very great. And entering into the sepulchre, they saw a young man sitting on the right side, clothed in a long white garment; and they were afraid. And he said unto them, 'Be not afraid: Ye seek Jesus of Nazareth, which was crucified: He is risen; He is not here: behold the place where they laid him. But go your way, tell his disciples and Peter that he goes before you into Galilee: there shall ye see him, as he said unto you.'

Can't you see it in your mind's eye…these ladies run to the disciples to tell them the good news! He's alive!! He's alive!!! He's risen from the dead!!!! Can't you see Peter, in the corner of the room, shocked, saying, what? What did you say? It's true! "Yes, He said to meet Him Galilee!" And Peter, who has been in the depths of depression for three days, stunned at the reality of the Resurrection, and almost encouraged, is once again plagued in his mind at his pitiful denial of Christ, and is dragged right back down into his pit of despair, and thought, "surely He doesn't mean for me to come…I denied Him three times, I cussed and swore…surely, surely He doesn't mean me!"

And the ladies said, oh, Peter, by the way…He mentioned you by name!!!

(Excuse me while I get Bapticostal!) Yes, He mentioned you by name! "He did? What'd He say?" He said, go tell the disciples…and Peter. Why did Jesus want to see Peter…to rebuke him? No, he wanted to <u>restore</u> him! And one of the sweetest scenes you'll ever see in scripture is Peter and Jesus, coming together, and Jesus hugging him and saying, Peter, do you love me? Not, "Peter, are you gonna cuss anymore?" No! He said, 'do you love me?' That's the real issue. If you're here today and you know you're a backslider, let me ask you, was there a time when you WERE right with Him? You see, the real question is not, are you gonna drink anymore? Curse anymore?…the real question today is "Do you love Him?"……… He loves you!

The napkin is still folded: He's still saving souls. He's still reclaiming backsliders! I heard about a little boy who had done something very naughty. His mother punished him. He was afraid his mother was still angry at him…in the kitchen there was a chalkboard on the wall where they wrote down phone messages. When no one was around, he wrote on that chalkboard, dear mom, if you forgive me, please wipe this out. He went to his room, and about an hour later returned, and to his surprise and joy that chalkboard had been completely erased!

Are you away from God right now? Bring your sins to the cross…

…Jesus will not rub them in, He'll rub them out!

If today you need to be saved, or you need to come BACK to God, I need to remind you there's coming a day when another supper will take place…it's called the marriage supper of the Lamb, and I have a feeling that at the marriage supper of the Lamb, that at the end of the meal, Jesus will stand at the head of the table, and He's going to wipe His fingers, mouth, clean His beard, and He's going take His napkin, and cast it aside…when that happens, it IS over! The last soul that's gonna be saved, has been saved. The last backslider that's going to come home has! I beg of you, don't wait 'til it's too late. Right now, the napkin is still folded! Remember the prodigal son…when he came home, his father welcomed him home with open arms! Today, Jesus is calling you home, the napkin is still folded!"

If you know Christ as your Lord and Savior together we are on the winning team as born again Christians. I love what that preacher of old said, "I have read the end of The Book and we win!" A woman wrote on the inside of her son's Bible as he went off to college, "Baby, this Book will keep you from sin or sin will keep you from this Book." It was my honor in 1999 to attend the Billy Graham School of Evangelism in Monterey, California.

Just shy of a thousand people were present at the conference and was informed I was one of the youngest to attend that year. One of the highlights for me was to hear in person one of my heroes of the faith, the late Dr. E.V. Hill and he preached the paint off the walls that night!

Dr. Hill talked about how God gave us power to 'Go into all the world and preach the Gospel.' Shortly after that sermon he passed away but I waited in line to thank him for his ministry and shared I had been a fan from afar for years and loved watching him minister on television.

Slightly nervous, I humbly asked him to kindly sign my Bible and he signed it writing his life verse. To this time, every time I approach the pulpit with God's Word in my hand I know that I am carrying greatness. Not just because of he who signed it but He (Jesus) Who sealed it with His Word and saving blood. We find boldness when bathed in the Bible and we cannot go wrong living for the Lord. The Bible says we can go boldly to the throne of grace and we need to stop acting like we lost when as kids of The King we already have won!

CHAPTER ELEVEN

CARRYING GREATNESS

Out of the gate, I want to remind you that each and every one of you reading this book and who ever breathed are invaluable in the eyes of God. You don't have to be around fame or hold fortune to be worth something. You are so valuable to God that on your behalf He sent His very and only son, Jesus to live a perfect life only to die in your place. No other leader or religion sent another to die in propitiation for our sin to bridge the gap for redemption. Honestly, none other is worthy or sufficient. The Bible in Acts 4:12 says it all (look it up).

Greatness is everywhere if we just pause long enough to look and see with a grateful heart. Pastor John Hagee, Senior Pastor of Cornerstone Church in San Antonio, TX once shared in a sermon the words on a sign affixed to a Houston Athletic Dormitory: "*I used to complain that I had no new shoes until I met the man who had no feet.*" Today, do you have the attitude of gratitude? True greatness is being grateful and gracious. It is an attitude found in many champions and worth more than the trinkets made by man.

One of the greatest sports illustrations on perseverance is NFL great and Hall of Famer, the late Walter Payton of the Chicago Bears. He was poetry in motion when he ran and when he hit opponents head on it was with enormous power as if a truck had run you over making it almost impossible for one man to tackle him. Payton was ill prior to a big game and just half hour before the kick off he was lying on the locker room floor wrapped in towels, shaking and sick with flu. Everyone told him to sit back, head home and go to bed but Walter wanted nothing to do with those instructions. With no time to spare, he suited up and broke the NFL single game rushing record of 275 yards! Over and over, when most would break I've seen others BREAK records. "Sweetness" knew intimately greatness and when he could hardly carry on his gift carried him. The late, great number 34 would say, "Suit up and don't quit!"

Greatness is also an attitude, ability and a craft that we have to be willing to work at and develop daily over and over without losing heart. Without question it is not going to be easy because honestly it will be at times downright discouraging, depressing and may lead to death. It will push you but also promote you but the key question is an age old one; are you truly willing to pay the price?

Both Presidents Lincoln and Kennedy were gunned down for speaking up and stepping out. However, monuments and Memorial Day parades are not made for critics or cowards but champions of Truth. Their examples remind us now that it is better to speak truth and die prematurely than live long sitting silently in the shadows or sideline.

God made you for His glory and to have a relationship with you. Jesus is not a professional Savior but a personal one and I love what Max Lucado wrote, "He would rather die for you than live without you!" It has been said, "The wealthiest place in the world is not in boardrooms or corporate America but in cemeteries." Sadly, many have taken their talents, gifts and dreams to the grave. Today is the time to develop those gifts and mentor those behind us. Keep in mind that not everyone will see your gift or respect your abilities. Quite honestly, it can be lonely at times when you realize you have an assignment. The weight can get heavy and the blessing is also a burden intertwined.

Just ask Joseph in Chapter Two. His brothers didn't love him but loathed him so much they wanted him dead. Your gift may cost you friends, family and bypassing fortune to live larger than just comfort and cash. We are created to honor God and bless others. Jesus couldn't do certain miracles in some towns because of their lack of faith and self righteous behavior. Don't let losers hinder you from winning at what God made you to be. Never become less in order for others to love you more. The problem with jumping through hoops for another is that you are the only one jumping! Live for an audience of One and if God be for you who can be against you?

One of the pitfalls of progress and promotion is that we get complacent. Worse, we can think that our success is all because of our labors and we had no help along the way. Wrong! It has been said, "If you see a turtle on a fence post it didn't get there by accident. Someone put him there!" One story that is engrained into my head is one I learned since visiting the majestic Niagara Falls this past summer while crisscrossing America. The sheer power of its rapids and the depth of those falls are almost unmatched. Truly, two atoms colliding in the sky didn't make that! The first three words of the Bible tell it all in Genesis Chapter One, "In the Beginning, GOD created the Earth."

May this story inspire you and humble us all to never take success for granted. Mr. Bobby Leach was the very first person to survive going over Niagara Falls in a barrel. The year was 1911, and this brother in a barrel dared to do something great. He wanted to graduate from mundane and do the mighty (even if it meant death). Niagara Falls received its name from an Indian term that means "The Strait." No, I am not referring to George Strait but the divide between the United States and Canadian border. The length of the brink at The Horseshoe Falls is a staggering 2,060 feet across and the drop is approximately 170 feet down! Couple that with over 600,000 gallons of water PER SECOND rushing over with such an enormous force that only God alone knows the exact power.

With skill within and grace above, Mr. Bobby Leach did in fact survive the ferocious falls of Niagara but would you like to learn how he died? No joke and not to be disrespectful, but Bobby died slipping on an orange peel! Definitely not making light of his death but we can learn so much from this life lesson. Regardless of what profession or ministry you are in now, be mindful that pride goes before the fall. Satan will give you a taste of success in public only to assassinate you in private.

Consider David who dared to dominate and defeat Goliath. Yes, he conquered Goliath with the Son but his sin conquered him with Bathsheba. Looking back, it was God and David as a team that toppled the giant by faith, but David derailed himself when he went alone in the flesh. My mentor and friend, Dr. Tim Lee, U.S. Marine Corps said, "You can get what you want but will lose what you had." It has also been said, "You can choose your sin but you don't get to pick your consequences."

Thank God for grace and SECOND CHANCES because truth be told we have all fallen short of the glory of God and made mistakes (Romans 3:23). True greatness comes from God's saving grace alone and apart from Jesus we are all doomed, dead and damned. Not glamorous, but Gospel Truth. If we are not careful, we can slip up over something we thought insignificant down the street. Why do most accidents happen less than five miles from our house? Perhaps because the area is familiar to us we have traveled down that road a thousand times, so we drop our guard. Complacency breeds catastrophe. It is imperative that we rely on the Lord for everything, both big and small because even honorable and humble people can slip up on silly peels.

Satan constantly is on the lookout, longing and would love to surprise us when we have our guard down. Especially after a big life or ministry experience because he is slick, slimy and that snake wants nothing more for souls to go to Hell and cripple, derail or tarnish those already heading to Heaven. If Satan can't get you unsaved he will make you feel unfit for future use. Read that line again because that may be the most powerful statement in the entire book. Most will fall in private way before tripping up publicly and may we humbly remember forever Mr. Leach who survived mighty Niagara but died on a little orange.

Visiting Niagara Falls literally took my breath away but if we elect to live life outside of the will of God that should take all our breath away. My buddy, Jamey Ragle is right when he said, "All of us are a step away from stupid." Any success apart from God's success is NO success at all.

Another pitfall to carrying greatness is not only becoming complacent but cocky and tempted to cut corners. In the early 1990's I was working as a summer intern at the United States Capitol. My duties primarily were raising the American flag over the roof next to the Rotunda. Spring 2014, marks the 150th anniversary of the dome on top of the United States Capitol and the Architect of the Capitol received the funds to refurbish it for future generations. Most folks start at the bottom in Washington but I was blessed to start at the top. Literally! You cannot get much higher than working on the roof of the Capitol Building and I loved every minute but it sure was hot in the summer! We had a string of 100 degree days and being two hundred feet above working on a copper roof it could easily be over 125 degrees on the roof.

Most folks don't like rain but when it did in the summer we would have to come down from the roof and do odd jobs inside the Capitol. Sometimes we would polish brass railings in Members Only elevators or set up platforms for a Presidential arrival. Other times we would vacuum congressional carpets or wash the larger than life statues in Statuary Hall or the Rotunda. If you ever have the privilege to tour the Capitol notice the shoes on those statues in the hallways. They shine differently because students when taking the tour rub the base of their feet and the oil from their fingers strips the coating on the statues. Honestly, my favorite assignment was one I was handpicked to do. Just below the staircase leading up to the Rotunda was a room called the crypt and now moved in a more public location inside the new billion dollar Capitol Visitor's Center. The crypt previously was a gated area that housed what I believe to be the most impressive artifact in the Congress.

Yes, I have seen the flag that flew over the Moon in the Sergeant at Arms Office and held the mace informing the world of our political power. It was my honor to have access to the Vice President's Ceremonial Office just off the Senate Floor which 99.9% of most folks have no clue it exists much less had the key to get in. Adjacent to the Vice President's Office is the President's Room which had drop dead gorgeous floor to ceiling size mirrors plated in gold with rich, red leather chairs and in the center of the room was the very table that President Abraham Lincoln signed his name granting freedom to shackled slaves on the Emancipation Proclamation. It was also the very holding room that modern day Presidents would relax until time to give their speech while in the Capitol. My father, Deputy Chief Frank Shelton, Sr. met The Reverend Billy Graham in that same room and was given his autograph by the world-wide evangelist.

But without question, my favorite attraction is one that most overlooked. Inside the gated area of the crypt was a two piece glass box that housed a black felt stand called the catafalque. This is the bier (stand) that supports the American flag draped coffin when a State Funeral is held in the Rotunda of the United States Capitol. The highest earthly honor is to have your funeral held in the Capitol and it takes an act of Congress to agree if the individual was worthy to be honored in death. The Lincoln catafalque was first used at his funeral in 1865. Most recently used on December 20, 2012 for Senator Daniel Inouye (D-Hawaii) whom it was my honor to meet and serve when I worked on the floor of the Senate in 1995. What are the odds and have had a connection to the first and most recent individuals to have lain in state? My ancestor with President Lincoln and Dad and I blessed to work alongside Senator Inouye.

One of the last assignments I had while working for the Capitol Police in the Office of the Assistant Chief was assisting in planning the funeral of our 38th President, Gerald Ford. He died on December 26, 2006 and I stepped out by faith to preach as an evangelist on July 27, 2007. It was my privilege to stand out in the heat in June 2004 to attend President Ronald Reagan's funeral and just as guards protected President Lincoln's even in death, who could forget the Secret Service escorting the casket to the awaiting hearse? That day even the black hearse had the presidential seal affixed to the door and President George W. Bush graciously loaned Air Force One, the Boeing 747 to transport Reagan's body. First Lady Nancy Reagan and family flew to Simi Valley, California where the funeral concluded at his Presidential Library.

President Reagan flew for years on the same Boeing 707 that flew Kennedy's body home from Dallas and took Nixon around the world. You could see that the plane was getting old. Towards the end of his presidency he lobbied Congress and was granted the appropriation for two brand new 747 aircrafts to be built to fly the president. It took nearly three years to make and his predecessor, President George Herbert Walker Bush (41) was the first to benefit from it. That is leadership right there. What will you leave behind to your predecessor and loved ones? Tragically, despite President Reagan ordering it he never flew on it alive but was carried on it in death. Ruth and I were blessed on December 18, 2013 to take a private tour at Andrews Air Force Base and thanks to two friends and the fine folks of the 89th Airlift we boarded the President's personal plane. What a treat it was to climb aboard "Air Force One" and spend nearly two hours on the Boeing 747 with the numbers 29000 on the tail with the American Flag on it. The fuselage and livery is painted white with the beautiful, baby blue color scheme that First Lady Jackie Kennedy helped design with the words "United States of America" are embossed in black.

If that plane doesn't give you goose bumps when looking at it one is either dead or not American. President Jimmy Carter, our 39th President was so excited the first time he flew on it shared this story, "I had just won the election to become President. It was an exciting time to say the least. President Gerald Ford was so gracious and he sent the plane to Albany, GA to take my wife and family to Washington for my inauguration. I was so excited to fly on "Air Force One" that en route to Albany to the airport that morning I realized half way there that we left my mother back in Plains, GA! We had to turn around and go pick her up and we were late getting to Washington."

Our Air Force One tour guide showed Ruth and I the four leather chairs in the rear of the plane that were removed to make room for President Reagan's casket. "Air Force One" not only transports presidents alive but can become a flying hospital equipped with a fully functioning emergency room aboard the plane should surgery need to be done at nearly 40,000 feet. In the corner of that mobile medical unit is a freezer containing the president's blood and every two hours as the world's most recognized aircraft is flying the plane is in constant communication with hospitals below who are on alert should the plane have to divert and make an emergency landing. The presidential plane is not only a flying White House or hospital but also acts as a flying hearse on rare occasions to retrieve the remains of their former top dignitary. Without question, the Air Force that day with the high honor of transporting President Ronald Reagan's casket and today with our Commander in Chief they continue to carry greatness. Not just the person or political party but the purpose and power that comes with the high office of our beloved nation.

Since Henry Clay in 1852, the United States Capitol Rotunda has been where a very select group of Americans have been honored by lying in state there. Some of those so honored have been eleven United States Presidents, military officers, an F.B.I. Director, Civil Rights icon, Ms. Rosa Parks and my good friend, Special Agent John Gibson who was killed in the line of duty while protecting House Majority Whip Tom DeLay (R-Texas) in 1998.

Agent Gibson was with the United States Capitol Police and we became friends half a decade earlier when I was employed in the Senate Post Office and later as a Doorkeeper on the Senate side. In 1993, I was contacted by the Senate Postmaster and called into her office and assigned to buy $15,000 worth of stamps at the D.C. Postal Distribution Center. The catch was she had staff entrust me, at barely twenty years old, all of it in CASH in a leather satchel. Two agents were assigned to walk beside and behind me to their unmarked police cruiser.

They transported me to the main mail distribution center in D.C. and I waited in line like everyone else but unbeknownst to everyone beside me and only the agents with me that I was holding a large amount of cash. That was a wild feeling and quite honestly, I didn't like the idea of holding all that money. I bought the stamps and with my agent friends adorning ear pieces and talking in their wrists, the officers followed me to the awaiting car. Folks on the street saw me with them and inquired was I a Congressman or a Senator? With a smile, Gibson and other agents at times went along and told them a junior senator. Those were good times and he was a class act. My heart stopped that day when while working in the Congressman's office I heard on the news that Special Agent Gibson had died. My mind raced to all our times together and we had a friendly competition as to who had the best joke of the day.

It is in my blood and I am positive that my ancestor who shared priceless moments joking with President Lincoln had a quick wit too. Most recently, it was discussed who may be eligible to be lain in state honored in the Capitol and The Reverend Billy Graham's name came up repeatedly but the family politely turned it down and have already made arrangements for a humble service at his library in Charlotte, North Carolina. He has been a friend and minister to the past twelve Presidents and I have always believed that God's power is greater than government's power.

Rev. Franklin Graham recently noted during Dr. Graham's 95th birthday celebration that on his father's tombstone he asked that it simply read: "*Billy Graham, preacher.*" That says it all and the greats indeed are gracious. He has preached to more people in person than anyone in history and three words sum up his life but in death he will hear seven, "Well done, thy good and faithful servant." Every time he got up to preach regardless if in a stadium or on a street, when he held up his Bible and proclaimed the Gospel he was carrying greatness and greatness will carry him Home. One of the greatest honors of my life is growing as friends with some of the Graham grandchildren and it is exciting to see them all serving in ministry.

While cleaning inside one of those rainy days in D.C., I was asked once again to return to the catafalque and clean it with a supervisor. We approached the gates and with key in hand opened the gates and as they slowly swung open we were tasked to Windex the glass case and then pull the two pieces apart. Gingerly after that we removed each case to the side and then vacuumed the black felt box that supported the caskets of heads of state from President Lincoln to JFK to Ronald Reagan and most recently Gerald Ford. It also supported the casket of my good friend, Agent John Gibson and his colleague, Officer Jacob Chestnut respectfully who was one month away from retirement when that sick assassin murdered him.

I had previously cleaned the catafalque probably half a dozen times in two years. It doesn't have to be done regularly but dust has a way to creep in the smallest crevices and this time my colleague tempted me with a proposition. He said, "Frank, no one is looking and the camera isn't recording us why don't you jump up and lay "spread eagle" on this. Immediately, I recalled Satan tempting Jesus on top of the Mountain in Matthew Chapter Four and asked Him to bow down to him and Christ refused. In my Spirit, as tempting as it was to be where greatness was I knew those men and few women died and deserved it and the honor was reserved for them. With time ticking, I picked up one of the glass cases and gently returned it in place to ensure a seal from dust until the next cleaning. It would have been dishonorable of me to do that for those honorable giants of freedom. While aboard "Air Force One" the host graciously asked if we wanted to sit one by one in the president's taupe leather chair in the front of the airplane; I admit it was tempting and one by one everyone else did but out of respect for the office and occupant I politely turned it down.

One of the tempting pitfalls of carrying greatness and promotion is not only cutting corners but consumed with the pull to benefit only self and neglect others. Having a special gift is like having a black belt in Karate. Sometimes you have to defend yourself but more than not you have to refrain from hurting those immature and crazy. If we don't use our gift for God and helping others, folks can get seriously hurt in the process. The Bible is clear: "To whom much is given much is required."

Keep in mind that jealousy is "lousy." It's no coincidence that the last five letters of jealousy spell lousy. Dogs don't bark and chase parked cars. They only run after those that are moving forward and Satan doesn't goes after the copper and bronze but silver and gold. Maybe that is why Olympians chase the first and not the latter. The greater your gift the more your critics will lash out but nothing is new under the sun and the heart is desperately wicked above all things. If we don't bridle our tongue, guard our hearts and refrain from releasing power in the flesh and not by faith, we all can get in trouble. Again, David killed Goliath by faith but almost got killed when operating in the flesh. God forgave but Bathsheba's husband was murdered. Sin always has consequences.

Michael Jackson about a year before his death was asked in a television interview: "Michael, you didn't have much of a childhood growing up. You were almost a man as a boy and at times acted like a kid as an adult. Under all that pressure and intense practice sessions if you could live all over again would you change anything?" The "king of pop" smiled and said, "No! I was born to be on stage." Michael knew that he was born to perform and his gift would bless millions. Greatness comes with a price.

During dinner one night, Meadowlark shared with me a story about his dear friend, Sammy Davis, Jr. He said, "Meadowlark, the world is my stage and the moment I walk outside I am expected to perform. If I don't feel up to it I stay home." The consummate showman knew the price and pain that comes with such a gift and when we give our gifts to God our burdens become light as we allow Him to carry us.

Some critics are confused fans. They study all day analyzing you but are too small to compliment you so their critique is their crazy way of giving you props. See it as a positive and not negative. Remember one day soon you will stand before Christ not crowds or critics. Keep your eyes on the prize and stay close and clean while moving forward by faith. It has been said, "Whatever we do for self will pass but what we do for Christ will last."

In 1995, while working as floor staff of the United States Senate I was invited to the Rotunda once again. In years past I had served behind the scenes and I recall in 1991 erecting the platform and placing plants on the stage and around the perimeter for the following day's remarks by President George H. W. Bush (41). A couple years later, I was asked to attend a conference featuring Grammy Winner Garth Brooks. I said, "Sure" and another Special Agent with the Dignitary Protection Detail of the U.S. Capitol Police whisked me down the hallowed halls. Honestly, I thought we would hear his speech and then have a brief second for a meet and greet and then return to my job.

The agent played a trick and instead of me sitting in one of the four hundred chairs placed in the Rotunda they had me come in another entrance and I realized we had a problem. In front of me was the crowd and to my horror I saw three television cameras with a red light on all of them telling this goofball that they were taping "LIVE." To my left speaking was Garth Brooks and to his immediate left were two others legends -- Grammy winners Michael Bolton and Kenny G! They asked me if I wanted to attend but I didn't ask to ambush their press conference.

Garth and his gang were there encouraging Congress on behalf of the National Endowment of the Arts and he was pleading with folks not to cut any funding. The country legend was wearing boots, jeans, denim shirt, ten gallon black hat and a big belt buckle that would make both Oklahoma and Texas proud! I was in trouble and I didn't ask to be on the scene much less on the stage and now he is staring at me. My political career just flew by my eyes and I knew we were in trouble.

To my right were the agents who played the little trick on me and gave the "thumbs up." Unfortunately, I can relate to another agent named Hill in Dallas when he signaled the "thumbs down" that President Kennedy was down and near death. Like Elvis, I am trying to 'leave the building' but I am stuck! When the speech was over hundreds rushed to meet him and I was trying to get out of Dodge (D.C.). Garth grabbed me and asked who I was and what I did? I told him the truth and he asked if I were a fan and I told him I was. He asked if any one of his songs encouraged me and I told him "Unanswered Prayers" was my favorite song of his. He no longer looked mad and said that was his most respected song and requested to sing on tour. Fortunately, we turned the corner and I love that chorus:

"Sometimes I thank God for unanswered prayers and remember when you are talking to the Man upstairs, just because He doesn't answer don't mean He don't care. It's just God's greatest gifts are your unanswered prayers."

I'm reminded "Happiness isn't getting what you want but wanting what you got."

Prayer is also not so much us talking to God but listening to His, still small voice. We need to adopt His agenda for our lives more than us demanding what we think we need. We sing God's praises in the victories but we show maturity and do well to sing, serve and shine for Him even in the valleys. One of my favorite jobs was being appointed in April 1995 by The Honorable Howard Greene (R) at the time who was the powerful Senate Sergeant at Arms and he tapped me to be one of the youngest aides in modern memory to work on the floor as a bi-partisan figure serving all 100 Senators. What a privilege it was to have a front row seat to serve and glean from some of the greatest orators of our time. I was only 23 years old at the time and half the day I would be on the Republican aisle and remaining portion of the day serving the Democrats. Senator Strom Thurmond (R-SC) was the President Pro Tempore and he was in his early nineties and I had the privilege to escort him daily on to the floor and up the rostrum. He was a living legend and quite feeble and he would hold on to my arm as I helped assist one of the most powerful politicians to ascend to his seat. He ran for President in 1948 and was the first southern senator to hire an African American on his staff.

Yes, he was holding on to me and the thought "Carrying Greatness" did bounce in my head like a kid on a trampoline but I knew even then it was really greatness carrying me.

During that time I had the pleasure to meet some wonderful people. To many those who serve in Congress are perceived as institutions but they really were for the most part dedicated individuals. It was a treat to talk daily with Senators and their staff. I carried a small black book and pen with me not to record any dirt but write down those who took time to say 'hi.' Common courtesy goes a long way in my book and you never know what a little encouragement can give to another. Yes, the greats are gracious. One memorable moment was the time that the liberal lion, Senator Ted Kennedy asked to borrow my Visa card. That was interesting! Looking back, I wish I thought quick enough to borrow his! A few months later we took a picture together by the Senate Reception area and before being appointed to work on the Senate floor ironically I delivered both his and Senator Strom Thurmond's mail when I was with the Senate Post Office a couple years before. Both of their offices were in the Russell Senate Office Building and fortunate to get pictures with both Senators and they both signed them personally. Regardless of politics it was an honor to be with both of those individuals. When the Senator from Massachusetts returned my picture he scribbled in his own handwriting, "*To my good friend, Frank Shelton. With very best wishes – Edward M. Kennedy.*" It was humbling that a kin to Camelot considered me a friend.

Right before Dad retired I asked Senate Majority Leader Bob Dole (R-KS) to graciously autograph a picture of the Capitol for my father. He did and that picture hangs proudly in the foyer of their home today next to the Supreme Court Justices who each personally signed their portrait for him as well. Dad was so blessed to have so many friends and accomplished so much in his law enforcement career on Capitol Hill. Dad told me years ago, "Frank, I can help you get in the door but it's up to you to get up and down the floors!" Then there was the time, Senator John Glenn (D-OH) and I talked on the Senate floor in 1995 about the soon to be released "Apollo 13" movie starring Tom Hanks. That was wild! Senator Glenn had been to the moon and I was a Senate space cadet! He had been in orbit and I was out to lunch.

We were blessed to meet everyone from janitors to presidents. God blessed me tremendously when I was able to grow as friends with two of the chaplains of the United States Senate. Both of them were Presbyterian ministers and the late Dr. Richard C. Halverson and Dr. Lloyd Ogilvie are two of the greatest men of God I will ever meet. I first met Dr. Halverson when I delivered his mail with the United States Senate Post Office in the early 1990's and he was the pastor to my godmother, Judy Henderson at Fourth Presbyterian in Chevy Chase, MD. Just three months ago, I preached at funeral honoring my late Aunt Bonnie Shelton's mother, Mrs. Barnes. She was 98 years old and her pastor for years was the late, great Peter Marshall, also a past chaplain to United States Senate. It was an honor to speak at her funeral and she was a saint. It was both a sad day and tremendous celebration when Dr. Halverson passed. Sad because we lost one of God's greatest generals serving in His Army but a party because he finally got to be Face to face with the One he lived and longed to see. I still have the VHS video of his funeral service in my bedroom and he touched thousands for God's glory.

Dr. Ogilvie and I became good friends and talked every single day before he opened the Senate in session with prayer. Previously before coming to the United States Senate as the chaplain he was President Ronald Reagan's pastor when "The Gipper" was still governor of California. Dr. Ogilvie was pastor of the well known Hollywood Presbyterian for several years and everyone from Hollywood to homeless loved him! Dr. Ogilvie gave me a copy of his book before it was released and autographed it for me and often would come on the back of the Senate Floor and sit next to me and we would quietly talk while they were in session. He was not only a great orator and teacher of God's Word but still a man of prayer. I saw him pray with his eyes closed and could tell when he was in private prayer while praying for our national leaders and nation. He epitomizes what it means to "pray without ceasing." I will never forget the time he personally tracked me down and invited him to be his guest at his weekly Bible studies in the Senate Office Building that he gave for staff. I have always said the greats are gracious and he is both.

One day he floored me and asked me out of the blue if I would drive him and accompany him as his guest to attend the National Prayer Breakfast and sit at his table. He was to speak that day along with the President of the United States of America (William Jefferson Clinton) but the keynote speaker was none other than Mother Teresa. A year later, I would become Congressman Hoyer's Special Assistant and full-time driver transporting him daily from his home to Capitol Hill and everywhere in between but this assignment in advance was something else. That invite was so kind of Dr. Ogilvie to want to share that with me and get to meet Mother Teresa but the truth is I didn't get the opportunity because I was sick and Mom advised me to not go for fear of getting one of the most respected women to ever live ill. My mother was right but that would have been a memorable moment to say the least.

Dr. Ogilvie is one of the most powerful preacher's I know and his voice is a blend of James Earl Jones and Dr. Adrian Rogers. Put them together in a blender and you have the voice of God. He was hands down the sharpest dressed man on Capitol Hill and many often mistook him for a United States Senator with his dapper suits, silk ties, matching handkerchief and trademark French cuff shirts and cufflinks. He was in a league all his own and he even brought me to his personal office to talk about my future in Washington and hinted about possibly bringing me on his staff. His wife was getting ill and he eventually left Capitol Hill and went back to the West Coast to minister to her. He had ministered to the world and some of the most influential people on the planet but like Christ willing to leave the masses and help individuals. Sometimes less is more.

The fact is greatness is all around and deposited in each and every one of us. I have seen it in Jamaica when speaking at Praisefest Ministries Cruise with a Cause crusade. That evening over 72,000 attended the festivals with many of the most recognized names in Christianity ministering. Earlier in the day, I was invited to speak at a public school and we met hundreds of students. This one young Jamaican boy came up to me and he was about nine years old. Our goal was to love them and encourage them while on the island to minister.

With several of my team members around me I reached out to shake his hand. However, he hesitated. It was awkward and then it seemed like eternity. He stared at my hand and then slowly moved up to my face and then looked me square into my eyes and after another pause he reached out and we finally shook hands. Then he said these words in his awesome accent, "Mon, you are the first white man I have ever shaken hands with." I was surprised, touched and humbled. In that moment it was a powerful connection and once again I just witnessed greatness.

Later that same night back on the ship, Ruth and I were dining with our dear friends, Michael Cramer of Florida and Ronnie "The Raven" previously mentioned from Missouri and two of my best buddies, Nikita Koloff and Lex Luger. Both of them are born again Christians, ministers of the Gospel and former World Wrestling Champs. Nikita was the "Russian Nightmare" and Lex still known around the globe as "The Total Package." I have had the honor to spend precious time with both of those Godly giants and we have ministered together in four countries and half a dozen states together. They have been to our home in Maryland and I have been fortunate to have dinner and spend the night in both of the champs' homes in North Carolina and Georgia.

During dinner, Lex was feeling fatigued and he had just suffered a stroke the year before and was still in pain at times. At times the champ relies on a walker to help him get around but on this night the former five time World Wrestling Champ was running extra low and slow. As we left our table on that gorgeous cruise somewhere floating at sea near Jamaica heading back to Miami, Florida, as soon as Lex got up we could tell in that moment he was going to need help. A couple steps were between our table and heading down from our section of the dining room as we headed towards the foyer to head out. Nikita asked me to grab one arm and he grabbed the other and together the former champ is now leaning on another champ (Nikita) and a chump (me).

Folks were watching us from neighboring tables but what an honor it was to assist a friend much less former champion. In the past and his prime, Lex had body slammed Hulk Hogan and pinned Ric Flair but now I found myself helping a friend needing a hand. Yes, the idea of "carrying greatness" traveled in my head while we walked towards his cabin room. The fact is Lex was known around by millions as the 'total package' but without Christ he would have never been the complete package! We both talked about that and filmed a video together and he wrote a chapter in my last book. That brother went from king of the ring to a lover of King of all kings!

A decade and half before when one of the greatest voices in Christianity was going through an extremely tough time and many wondered if he would ever sing again, God impressed deeply in my heart to reach out and correspond with him. For nearly a decade, the Lord led me to write letters of encouragement, hope and Scripture and while doing it I knew with the aiding of the Holy Spirit displaying class, compassion and modeling the heart of Christ in another's storm enabled us to lighten the load together. At that moment, God writing through me while reaching out to him together we were "carrying greatness." Praise the Lord, that precious brother is back stronger and singing better than ever. Thank God for grace and I learned that when we love on folks in their valleys they won't forget us when they get back to the mountain top.

Greatness abounds and is all around. Regardless if it is turning the corner in a relationship or witnessing the light bulb go off in a classroom when a student finally gets it that is greatness. The child from a broken home who has been knocked down and kicked around and yet won't give up, we find greatness. When it would be easier to hoard our resources but we share with others, indeed is an attribute of greatness. When youth stay inside, obey their guardians and do their homework instead of running the streets, stealing cars and causing trouble that is pursuing greatness. As a spokesperson for Compassion International while in Guatemala I got to meet the girl that Ruth and I are blessed to sponsor monthly. Honestly, I wish I could have brought all the hurting and destitute home to help them find love and support. What broke my heart was to see children playing on top of trash dumps searching for food and passing time. Our team got to go into schools and connect with the students. We played games with them and sang songs and tried to befriend as many as we could. Today, Compassion has helped over a million people because of faithful contributions from folks supporting the precious children in multiple nations. Many of the children have grown up and graduated from college because someone else cared. Both displayed greatness, the giver and the recipient of the gift. When I lifted them above my head and heard them laugh with the largest smile possible I knew I was holding greatness. When public school bus drivers make minimum wages transporting our most prized possessions they are indeed carrying greatness. Our children are winners today not tomorrow! It is astonishing to me that we pay millions for athletes but next to nothing for our soldiers, policemen, teachers and bus drivers. Our priorities are askew.

At times greatness is not always obvious at the start but in the end is evident. We learned that with the Cherry Blossoms but also consider the Wright Brothers from Kitty Hawk, N.C. On December 17, 1903 they blocked out their critics and kept dreaming and daring while designing that first flight that flew for a whopping 18 whole seconds! While most sat on their sofa those Wright brothers had the "right stuff." Ironically, it was exactly a century, decade and a day later on December 18, 2013 that Ruth and I boarded "Air Force One" at Joint Andrews AFB in Maryland. Had those brothers not stuck with the stuff and chased their dreams we wouldn't had been on that majestic airplane. Their persistence has carried millions of passengers including presidents along for the ride every since.

Ponder Rudolph the Red Nosed Reindeer from that children Christmas classic. At first he was picked on and bypassed by his friends because he was different. Initially the other members made fun of him but what some saw as trash, the Master saw as treasure. Santa promoted him to the lead the way and greatness is often found in obscure packages. Talk about a night light! It was his red nose that carried Santa to deliver the goods! No, I am not implying that Santa is our Savior but Saint Nicholas was certainly the leader of that pack.

A week before going to London for the 2012 Olympic outreach as a chaplain I got a direct message on Twitter from Maryland native, former gold medalist and World Boxing great "Sugar Ray" Leonard. The champ (Leonard) asked me to extend his best wishes with a member of Team USA boxing team to let them know he was in the proverbial corner. That was considerate of him and I knew with that message I was entrusted to carry greatness. He has been gracious and kind and we have followed each other on

Twitter for several years now. Often when I am scheduled to preach where he used to train in Maryland I would give him a shout out. He is often kind to respond. Two years ago, I was the winner of his "Real Steel" movie essay and he picked me first place and the award was an autographed DVD from him of the Hugh Jackman boxing hit. Many are unfamiliar that it was Leonard who served as the fight consultant and coordinator for that movie to make the boxing fights look authentic. We met briefly when I was sixteen in Maryland and his son attended the same basketball camp my brother, Matt and I did. Ray was then and still one of my heroes. His fights against Hearns, Hagler and Duran are for the ages! I am looking forward to actor, Usher playing Ray in the upcoming Hollywood movie "Hands of Stone."

It is sure to be a 'hit!"

As a child my parents took me in 1981 to watch Muhammad Ali fight in a charity boxing match in Washington, D.C. In front of a crowd of several thousand organizers had a free raffle to give away the champ's Everlast trunks, robe, boxing gloves and size fourteen white shoes that he wore in the fight. My mother actually won the white Everlast boxing shoes that he wore in that fight and three decades later we still have them. Every time I hold Ali's iconic shoes in my hands I know they are special. On a side note, Sugar Ray Leonard gave one of his championship boxing belts to Nelson Mandela and said he was the "People's Champion." That was very gracious once again of the champ (Ray) but the true King of the Ring is Christ. He is the real Peoples' Champion.

Closing out this chapter, I will leave you with this powerful point. After midnight on the morning of May 2, 2011 twenty-three SEALs and their interpreter launched the raid on the top floor bedroom of Osama bin Laden's residence in Abbottabad, Pakistan. The highly trained SEAL Team 6 after flying in by helicopter of which one was destroyed upon arrival penetrated the compound, quickly killed two of the al Qaeda leader's assistants and while working their way upstairs adorning night vision goggles shot and killed the terrorist who had inflicted so much harm around the globe. Ironically, he didn't put up much of a fight when it was his time to go. Like many thugs they die cowardly at the end. Guilt gives up but grace doesn't quit.

Less than a week after the raid, members of the SEAL team who CARRIED out the mission briefed President Obama. According to sources present in the room the Commander-in-Chief asked to meet and shake the hand of the SEAL who shot Osama bin Laden. It was noted that they didn't move or say a word. CNN reported in an article the team commander then replied, "Mr. President, respectfully we will not tell you. If you took one person out of the puzzle, we wouldn't have the competence to do the job we did, everybody's vital. It's not about the guy who pulled the trigger to kill bin Laden, it's all about what we did together."

The fact was each of those trained SEALS individually were the elite of special ops in the world. They were prepared as the best and ready for the worse and on that assignment each of them willing, ready and able to pull the trigger. It was indeed a team effort and without question, each of them carried greatness to their target and completed their assigned task. They had it and you do too! As they raced to the awaiting helicopter the SEALS carrying bin Laden in the body bag were not carrying greatness but garbage. Here was a man made by the Creator of the world like everyone else and he had potential, power but threw it all away on hurting instead of helping others, and he failed to honor God. After the CIA confirmed that the body was in fact bin Laden, they took his remains to sea and threw him overboard and fed him to the sharks.

Last month, the United States Men's Hockey Team took the ice to face the Russians during the 2014 Winter Olympics in Sochi. I was up first thing in the morning to watch praying for another "miracle on ice." NBC once again elected to air the match on tape delay but I hate to catch things second hand and was fortunate to find it LIVE on real time on another channel. It was about eight in the morning and my family was still in bed on a lazy Saturday morning.

Honestly, I was feeling good about our chances and I was reminiscing about my recent Olympic experience two years before in London and already excited about going to Brazil for 2016 Olympics serving as part minister and motivator. My mind came back to the game at hand and I had a few friends in Sochi and I was praying for their safety and that God would use them for His glory.

As I was on the couch cheering for the red, white and blue my cell rang. As I glanced it read my sister's cell and I don't often hear from her first thing on a Saturday morning. I answered and what I heard next was slow motion. She was crying so hard I could not make out our conversation. In between the sobs I asked her to repeat it and when I finally pieced it together it was surreal.

The big game I was watching seemed so small and now I was pulling for TEAM USA like never before. Aaron Torian may not be familiar to you but he is family to us. I met him a quarter of a century ago and he is my brother in law's best friend and my nephew's godfather. Aaron was in the United States Marines Corps and he did not one, two, three, four or five but SIX tours overseas fighting for freedom. He was named "MARINE OF THE YEAR" two years before and was Special Ops making him the best of the best. My sister relayed to me that Aaron's wife had just got word that he hours before while in Afghanistan was hit by an IED and blew off both of his legs.

My sister was asking me to pray to God and that he would live. They were trying to stabilize his body and were en route to take him to Germany. We began to pray and call friends across America to intercede and the Olympics were such a blur on the big screen. Immediately, my mind raced to when we first met. Aaron was a gifted athlete and larger than life. The only thing bigger than Aaron's muscles was his heart and smile. When he walked in the room you sensed someone special was "in the house." He loved family, friends and possessed great faith in God and loved our country. He saw his service as a calling and he answered. Three hours later my sister informed me that MSgt Aaron Torian didn't survive and they were making plans to fly his remains to Dover, Delaware and my sister and her husband were going to be there personally with Aaron's wife to receive his body back on USA soil. The military calls it a 'dignified transfer.' When the plane landed at Dover AFB they slowly, delicately and reverently pulled out his American Flag draped casket as soldiers and generals saluted while his wife and our family with blurry vision welcomed home not only a hero but a dear friend.

The next day, I was honored to be a guest on "HANNITY" in the Fox News studio in New York City and the invite to appear had come in three weeks before. The next day, I flew to Houston, Texas to speak three days in a row in the Lone Star State and after flying home to Baltimore, Maryland late on Tuesday evening it was my privilege to be with the family as Aaron was buried with full military honors at Arlington National Cemetery.

He was a hero in every sense of the word and generals to janitors came to pay their respect. At the reception a familiar face walked in and it was none other than Lt. Col Oliver North and he spoke at the funeral. When a hero calls you a hero it is evident you are a hero. "Ollie" is also a Fox News contributor and twice he returned to Afghanistan with the Fox film crew and who served as his guard and body man was none other than "Marine of the Year" and our very own, "T" short for MSgt Aaron Torian.

My Dad had met Colonel North over two decades ago on Capitol Hill and it was good for them to reunite. I shared with Colonel North a quote from President Ronald Reagan, "Millions wake up every single day wondering if they make a difference. The Marines don't have that problem."

Lord knows Aaron made a HUGE difference! As the Marines carried one of America's best and our dear family friend to rest without question I knew instantly they were carrying greatness. When the seven Marines shot three times each for the 21 gun salute I knew they were paying respect to greatness. When the lone bugler played "Taps" on the snow covered hill at Arlington with tears rolling down his cheeks like Niagara Falls I knew he was honoring greatness. On bended knee when one of the distinguished Marine honor guard presented the flag folded like a football on behalf of the President and a grateful nation I knew they were thinking of greatness; not only Aaron whom was great but our beloved country.

Please pray for Aaron's family as he lives behind a wife and three small children. No, freedom is not free and all gave some but some gave all. Recently, I was pulling for TEAM USA and now in more ways than one. I am convinced they beat the Russians that day in the preliminary game and won for Aaron. The real heroes in life don't wear capes nor memorialized in halls of fame but folks like Aaron whom stare fear in the face and smile even in death. We lost one of the greats and God bless Aaron, his family and these United States of America. We are all better because of his sacrifice. Thanks to God's grace we both serve in His Army and we will see him again. #SemperFi

Bin Laden was a disgrace and Aaron was saved by grace. We honor the honorable but discard the dishonorable. We remember those who dared to dream and do right but forget the nightmares. Those who die without Christ will soon realize that Hell was no joke and certainly no party. We will find no beer, bikinis or bikes below. Heaven will be a marriage but Hell is a mirage. Mark this down -- there is no honor in Hell nor will you find any Award Ceremony outside of Heaven.

My pastor shared in the pulpit years ago of a submarine that was rammed by another ship and sank in the north eastern part of America. Rescue was now impossible and a diver was sent to see if there was any life aboard the sunken vessel. In the depth and darkness of the ocean a lone diver placed his ear against the hull of the sub and to his surprise heard a faint tap. Quickly, he made note of the dashes and dots and decoded the message: "Is – there— any—hope?" With a sunken heart he tapped back to the survivors in that sunken ship: "Hope – in—God—alone." The message of that diver is the mission for every born again believer today. Yes, we carry greatness but truth be told those apart from the saving grace of God to this day carry a sin virus with a death warrant and only hope is in Jesus. The Christian will be awarded and rewarded for their labors but the saint or sinner cannot be saved by their works.

Of all the attributes of greatness the greatest of them all is God's grace. It is not something we earn or purchase but can receive freely. We cannot add to it or subtract from it and it's because of God's sacrifice not in our service. We find them in His merits not our mercy. If we miss out on God's grace in life we miss out on everything in our death. You can get everything else right but if you died without God's grace you had it all wrong. The most recognized song known to man is "Amazing Grace." John Newton wrote that classic and the words are below.

"Amazing Grace, how sweet the sound,
That saved a wretch like me....
I once was lost but now am found,

Was blind, but now, I see.

T'was Grace that taught...
my heart to fear.
And Grace, my fears relieved.
How precious did that Grace appear...
the hour I first believed.

Through many dangers, toils and snares...
we have already come.
T'was Grace that brought us safe thus far...
and **Grace will lead us home**.

The Lord has promised good to me...
His word my hope secures.
He will my shield and portion be...
as long as life endures.

When we've been here ten thousand years...
bright shining as the sun.
We've no less days to sing God's praise...
then when we've first begun.

Amazing Grace, how sweet the sound,
That saved a wretch like me....
I once was lost but now am found,
Was blind, but now, I see"

When our time is up it will be that same grace and only that grace that will carry the child of God Home. Those who possess grace will be transported to Heaven and unfortunately all the rest will be dumped and duped in Hell. Not glamorous but the Gospel Truth. Carrying greatness is one thing but having grace carry you is everything.

This is our one shot to get it right and the Bible doesn't promote reincarnation but a resurrection and once you receive that, you will have the revelation to be the resolution to bless others. True greatness is not a possession or purpose but knowing the Person who makes life possible.

Chapter Twelve

Sharing Greatness

In the previous chapter I shared carrying greatness but this one focuses on sharing. If you care than you will share. One of my favorite stories is entitled "Stranded Starfish." The story goes that a young boy was on a beach picking up and tossing starfish in the ocean. A person walking by asked: "What are you doing?" The lad replied, "The tide is moving out and if I don't toss the starfish back to sea they will die." The man replied: "Why waste so much energy on something that is a waste of valuable time? Son, there are literally thousands of beaches and millions of starfish around the globe. How can you make a difference?" Looking at all the stranded starfish on the beach he resolute and undeterred picked another starfish in his hand and replied, "Mister, you are right. I cannot reach them all but to this stranded starfish it will make all the difference!"

Today, millions upon millions of stranded starfish souls are still stuck in society's sin sick shore waiting to hear of the saving Savior and compassionate Christ. Will the real men and women of God stand up and care enough to dare to share the glorious Gospel and toss them into our Savior's saving sea of salvation. Will you care enough for their eternal fate to point others to Jesus? Our job is to not clean them first but communicate in Christ-like words and deeds about the saving grace of God and watch Him pick them up, dust them off and redeem them from sinners to saints and become kids of The King. I am convinced that saved people want to see people saved. I love what D.L. Moody said, "Lord save the elect and elect some more!" God did not die for the few but for all who will call upon the Name of the Lord. Sadly, most

Christians have enough of Jesus to get them to Heaven but apparently not enough of Christ to keep others from Hell. You cannot take possessions to Heaven but you can sure take people with you! It is a travesty to enter Heaven empty handed.

We are compelled to win souls and a disciple will never become one unless a decision was made first. The evangelist, pastor and Christian must all do their part to help folks grow in maturity and grace. We do better to work together. The Scriptures are clear, "He that winneth souls is wise (Proverbs 11:20)." Jesus said, "You MUST be born again." It wasn't a suggestion but a statement from the only Savior known to mankind. The Bible says in Daniel 12:3 "And they that be wise shall shine as the brightness of the firmament; and they that turn many to righteousness as the stars forever and ever." In Proverbs 14:25: "A true witness delivereth souls: but a deceitful witness speaketh lies." We are not instructed to grow a church but help expand the Kingdom. God is not coming back for a brick building but blood bought believers. Those totally in tune to God desire daily to see someone (if not EVERYONE) come to Christ.

The term 'soul winner" to some may be a complaint but to Christ and the committed Christian is a compliment. That would be an awesome epitaph on a tombstone: "Frank Shelton, soul winner!" Jesus does the saving but we better do some sowing. The sole focus of ministry should be souls. Yes, we are to make disciples but a decision precedes the practice of discipleship. Like that old hymn: "I have DECIDED to follow JESUS!" Seeing souls saved should not be secondary but primary in church, ministry and our personal walk with Christ. Saved people should want to see people saved. Not just clergy but Christians! What good is doing missions if it doesn't lead to The Great ComMISSION?

My opening statement at the beginning of this book in the section entitled word to the wise, "Just because one is smart doesn't mean they are wise." One could have more degrees than a thermometer but may our heart burn more than our head knowledge. Don't let your theology hamstring you from doing what God has commanded us to do. You will have no excuse when standing before Christ. We are commanded to not only keep the faith but share it. When carrying greatness we are not only instructed to share Christ but class in the process. Legalism is high on the law and low on love.

One of my favorite all-time illustrations is about a young Christian that was at a state college. He was on fire for God and lived for the Lord. Whenever he saw people he would share the love of Christ and on occasion share a Scripture verse to encourage them. A group of athletes approached him and said, "We realize you mean well saying hi and acting like Christ to everyone but you need to chill out a tad." At that moment, an attractive girl walked by and the football players said to him, "You see that girl there?" He replied, "Yes." They said, "Don't waste your time on her. She is too far gone! She is gorgeous but her reputation is horrible. She has slept with half the football team and rumor has it she is sleeping with one of the coaching staff. She is too far gone and can't be saved." His heart sank and as they left he said a silent prayer for them and her because no one is beyond the saving reach of God.

Whenever he crossed paths with her he always smiled and was kind and Christ-like. At the end of the semester he was getting ready to leave for the summer and a knock was on his dormitory door and he swung it opened and before him was the very girl that the football players told him to give up on. She stared silently at him for a minute and then tears welled up in her eyes saying these words that minister to me deeply still two decades after first hearing this true story. She said, "I'm not sure if you know my story or my reputation. Years ago, before I strayed my momma always told me about a man who walked the Earth filled with kindness, compassion and forgiveness." Through blurry vision she said, "I am coming by today to ask you are you that Man?" With tears in his eyes he said, "No, I am not Jesus but will be glad to introduce you to Him and the girl who was heading for Hell because of God's grace and the witness of a Christian immediately became a daughter of the King!" If you learn one thing from this book is that JESUS SAVES!

Today, at 41 years old and a month away from turning 42, I would like to share about 43. No, not my age but two class acts! Over the years, I have witnessed something early on and it's my burning desire to live and leave. Some things are taught but the best things are caught. However, we can also learn a valuable lesson when we or another drop the ball or in this case miss the kick.

In case you are related to Rip Van Winkle and were asleep during arguably the greatest college football game in modern history you would know what transpired recently in the Alabama vs. Auburn rivalry. For starters, Nick Saban and his team rarely lose but have now lost twice recently to their arch rivals. On November 30, 2013 during the Iron Bowl after already missing a couple field goals opposed to the 'Hail Mary' the legendary coach sent his field goal unit out to attempt a FIFTY SEVEN yard kick to win the game. With only a second remaining the commentators were surprised to see Alabama setting up to kick rather than attempting a throw deep or even taking a knee. Alabama's kicker, Cade Foster is number 43 for the reigning national champions.

Despite Foster giving it his best effort, the unthinkable happened. Auburn with a newer coach without legendary status was more prepared on this play and sent a player in the end zone just in case the kick missed. The odds of missing it were pretty good (even NFL kickers would struggle with that distance); but for the ball to actually fall short into an awaiting player's hands is just shy of the odds of being hit by lightning. Keep in mind the end zone is sixty yards wide and add those odds with the fact that he was prepared to field it as if a punt return only to run 109 yards for a touchdown without being touched was nothing short of winning Maryland's recent Mega Million lottery! Let's not forget this is not against a lackluster junior varsity squad but against the best college football team in America. In this case, lightning struck twice and Alabama went from "Roll Tide" to unfortunately roll tears and the Auburn Tigers won. Cue up the Rocky III soundtrack because on that night Auburn had Alabama's number and like Sly Stallone and tunnel vision had "Eye of the Tiger."

Yes, as a resident of the Great State of Maryland, I pull for most local sports, but in college football Alabama is my team of choice. Today, I am blessed to call several of their past national championship team players and their families as friends while serving on the board with Tuscaloosa's based Praisefest Ministries "Cruise with a Cause." That night following the game, I called my buddy, Evangelist Randy Hogue of Cullman, Alabama who loves Auburn and immediately he hit me with this joke: "Frank, what does an Auburn fan say to any request of an Alabama fan?" I said: "No idea." He replied laughing, "Give me ONE SECOND!" Nothing like encouragement after a loss!

All that was the back story but this is what transpired next. Fights broke out. One Alabama fan watching the game with friends at home was so distraught over the loss that she picked up a loaded firearm and shot and killed another because she didn't think in her estimation that she was a true fan or was grieving hard enough that Auburn won. God help us! Then for the next couple days (non-stop) they attacked the poor kicker who missed. First, how many of the critics under that pressure with multiplied millions watching would have made it much less on an empty field with nobody but God in Heaven and a field goal post on Earth. Very few!

Secondly, some went to Twitter and personally called out and attacked the kicker verbally. One said, "Drink bleach," another said, "Go kill yourself," while one tweeted, "I know where you live and I am coming over to kill you!" Wow!! All this over a game!!! This is where you can insert "Get a life!!!!" Not to the kicker who missed the field goal but to so many of us who missed the point. Anyone can be a critic but it takes class to create and complete the task at hand. Personally, until we can kick a fifty yarder through the uprights we don't deserve to criticize. Ironically, those who are able to kick a fifty yarder usually refrain from criticizing.

You have heard of the expression, "The Good, Bad and Ugly" but today I gave it to you in reverse order. I shared the ugly first (murder is worse than slander but not by much) and then the bad but now saved the best (good) for last. Fox News reported despite all the hate mail, barrage of negativity, constant criticism out of nowhere appeared hope and encouragement. The former leader of the free world, President George W. Bush (43) reached out to the Alabama kicker (43) who missed the big kick. It is amazing what one kind word, letter of encouragement or a proverbial pat on the back can do for someone who is down and out. Regardless of your politics, it was a class act for the president to reach out.

Notice the date of the letter the former President wrote to the kicker. He penned it (December 3, 2013) not long after the game. When you have a chance to encourage another you shouldn't wait forever to do it because they need it now, not next year. Plus, their tomorrow may not come. As I write this chapter, a well-known pastor from Florida recently committed suicide this week. It saddens me to wonder if anyone reached out to him and I wish more would have shown class and compassion to him in his time of need. Secondly, if anyone was busy and had a free card to be exempt from picking up a pen and paper it was the former President. Our excuses go out the window when you realize his responsibilities.

Despite not spending as much time in Washington lately his calendar is still quite full. Within days of this letter he flew at midnight to Washington, DC from Dallas and he and his wife, Laura boarded "Air Force One" with President Obama. For the next 45 hours he traveled half the globe to pay respects to Nelson Mandela's family at the funeral. President George W. Bush even gave a speech in another nation while the world's most recognized Boeing 747 was refueling. Yes, President Obama spoke at the funeral in Africa but very few knew President Bush spoke overseas en route home to the United States. As an occasional White House press correspondent I am privy to POTUS daily schedule in advance, guidance and press briefings. During that historic trip while receiving almost hourly updates I learned almost in real time that even the pool traveling on the historic flight had no idea that Bush (43) snuck off to speak and were astounded! God only knows how much he accomplished in the last week that no one notices. Then again, leaders like President Bush didn't get to the top in their respective fields by accident. Leadership is never lazy.

Just as important, we can all relate and sympathize with others more in setbacks than in success. The second sentence of the note written by Bush to Cade Foster is remarkable because the President talks about him personally knowing about loss, hurt and defeat. It was because of his past pain that he could offer advice on perseverance in the present. President Abraham Lincoln suffered intense dark depression but was not just the Commander in Chief but the consummate Cheerleader in Chief constantly pushing for and promoting others. Our pain today can be a form of ministry and encouragement to another tomorrow.

Lastly, those that have already been to the mountain top desire nothing more to help encourage others in their temporal valley to move forward in their future. When you have been with the best you want others to be blessed. It is no longer competition but all about camaraderie. Who would have thought that Alabama's biggest fan would have been a Texan?

Ironically, Meadowlark's number in basketball is 34 and when you reverse the numbers its 43. When we take a long look in the mirror we all would do well to resemble 43 too. When Meadowlark cheered Tim Tebow in his success and President Bush encouraged Foster in his setback, both men showed class and compassion. Indeed, in more cases than not the greats are gracious. We may not all be known world-wide or be an official "globetrotter" but we can exude class and practice compassion. It takes maturity to root for another in their success and it takes just as much class and leadership to risk reaching out when others are hurting. I have learned like that REM song, "Everybody Hurts" and unfortunately not everyone is helping. In closing, the next time you see someone lose or succeed may we resemble winners and cheer them on.

Another attribute of sharing greatness is not only considering others before self but desiring to open doors for another. We have talked about sharing Christ and class but we must also extend compassion. A dirt poor boy from Tupelo loved to hear the all night Gospel concerts in neighboring Memphis. Some of the Southern Gospel's finest would sing to a packed crowd at the legendary Ellis Auditorium. A sixteen year old, unknown Elvis Presley fell in love with the songs and was mesmerized how the singers could sing harmony and that was when he first heard J.D. Sumner sing bass. Those concerts were so popular that folks drove from far and wide to attend and crowds grew above 5,000! Elvis would scratch and save for a ticket and became friends with his heroes and immediately began to dream of singing one day on stage! Elvis soaked in all the spiritual songs and borderline idolized the singers. J.D. Sumner is in the Guinness Book of World Records for having the lowest bass voice ever recorded. He was not only a giant in height but Elvis' hero.

On one occasion, J.D. noticed that the young boy who had been attending the sings so faithfully was absent. Then, the next time, he was back. When he had the opportunity to speak to Elvis, J.D. asked him where he was at the last concert and why he hadn't attended? Elvis embarrassingly replied that he didn't have enough money for a ticket. J.D. told him he wouldn't need any money from that point on. Sumner said, *"You just come to the stage door and I'll let you in for nothing"*. And that's the way it remained. Later, J.D. said, 'About the next thing I knew he was letting me in his stage door'. It was the beginning of one of the most enduring friendships of Elvis Presley's life. It has been said what you do for others God will do for you! Are you noticing a trend here? President George W. Bush at the top of his game reached out to another down and out. J.D. Sumner, a musical legend at the top of his game reached out to an anonymous kid who would later rock the world in music. The greats are gracious and you don't have to be the best to help but we can sure act like it when we do. Diana Ross was right, "Reach out and touch somebody's hand. Make this world a better place, if you can."

Without question, I also believe the doors we open for others the Lord very well may open for us. Regardless, of what vocation or industry you are in the one thing we could use more of is, service and stellar attitude. We live in a 'me' first society and it's tempting to buy the lie 'I better get mine first before someone else beats me to it.' That includes approaching doors, pole position at a red light, or cutting in line for a ride at the amusement park or buying groceries. Have you ever seen the customer with 54 items in a ten item or less line? #Hello

Selfishness is one of the most disgusting deodorants. In ministry, Jesus calls us to be servants and stewards even before speakers. A communicator without the "fruit of the spirit" is like wearing a silk suit with tie and cufflinks on the beach reading the paper. One may look good doing it but completely out of place and worse irrelevant.

In life, I met many who promote Christ but don't always pause and open doors for others (both literally and vocationally). Life lesson: Every door has a hinge. It cannot swing open wide if it didn't have a hinge. Doors to a janitor closet and even the curved doors opening the Oval Office have hinges. We need more folks to resemble that little device because our potential and even future promotion may HINGE on helping others. My motto is when approaching a door is this. I know by God's grace I was going to open it anyways – WHY NOT OPEN IT FOR OTHERS in the process? We need an open door policy and we should be an open door people as born-again Christians.

You may recall in a previous chapter, I was a doorkeeper at the United States Capitol for the Senate for two years (1994-1995). I adored that job. Get it – a DOOR that job! It was a privilege to hold the door and meet countless people in the process and interact with everyone from dignitaries to homeless, professional athletes to spouses of United States Senators. Plus, the Biblical admonition is true – "The greatest among you is the servant." Consider the doormen at fancy hotels who work for someone bigger than self and they have a chance to connect with all walks of life. It's amazing what a single act of kindness can do. Today, we need more service with a smile. By doing the little things big it can not only make a difference but make someone's day. The blessing is being the blessing! I would rather be a doorman for Divinity than be waited on by the Devil. No higher calling than being a servant of the Most High God. Service is a form of ministry to humanity. You may not have opportunity today to open door for a big job or television show but you can certainly hold that elevator that was closing on the single mother with a baby in her arms. Ministry is not just to the masses but ministering to individuals because everyone needs a helping hand.

In this chapter, I will leave you with two amazing examples of sharing greatness. One is political and other is personal however both are powerful. If anything is missing in modern day society it is teamwork. Being around Washington, D.C. my entire life you may be considered a political insider when you not only know the names of nationally known politicians but they and some of their security detail know you! My Aunt Barbara Shelton went to the senior prom at Suitland High School in the late 1950's with former House Majority Leader Steny H. Hoyer (D-MD). Congressman Hoyer represents my hometown and he has been a friend of the family for decades. My cousin married former House Majority Leader Dick Armey's son (R-TX) and at one time was one of the most powerful men in Washington. It's also a treat to reunite with some of his family when back in the Lone Star State. Honestly, I am uncertain if any other family in America has been linked to two House Majority Leaders of two different political parties.

Over the years, I have been blessed to see some pretty amazing things and other than sitting at an inauguration watching the transfer of power, especially of two different political parties one of my favorite things to witness is the transporting of an American President. In the past I was honored to fly four times on the Boeing 757 known as "Air Force Two." It is rare to fly on "Air Force One" and even more rare to fly on "Marine One." My Aunt Barbara Shelton (now deceased) married Joe Quinn from the Eastern Shore of Maryland and he is a well respected businessman and CPA. He ran for Congress in the late 1970's and lost by a minimal margin but was invited to fly on Marine One with the President who gave a speech in his honor at a campaign stop.

Regardless of where the Marine Corps pick up the President they carry the leader of the free world on one of several dark green helicopters with white letters "United States of America" to the awaiting plane on the runway. It is quite a sight to behold when you see two of the world's most iconic and powerful modes of flight transportation working together side by side to get the job done. Even more impressive is that they both desire that the other succeeds. Teamwork often includes two distinct groups united in one common goal. The U.S. Marines and U.S. Air Force respectfully have two totally different job descriptions but when it comes to transporting and ensuring the safety of their Commander in Chief they know their role and do whatever it take to be successful in furthering their mission and his agenda.

As soon as the President disembarks the Marine helicopter (HMX-1) he is greeted by the commander of the military base and escorted to the awaiting Air Force airplane. As soon as one mission ends the second starts racing down the runway. It is the passing of the baton similar to John the Baptist announcing in advance the coming of Jesus, The Christ. My question is if the military can work together today for a common good at the highest level of government why do so many presently in either ministry or secular business strike out? President Ronald Reagan had a sign in the Oval, "It's amazing what one can accomplish if you don't care who gets the credit." Pride kicked Satan out of Heaven and that same arrogance will hinder many others while on Earth. More than ever we need a team spirit and willing to sacrifice ego to benefit others. Never let your insecurity rob another of their destiny. This example is powerful but the last is personal.

On another note, you may recall my pastor, Rev. Marvin Harris from our last book we co-wrote, <u>Blessedness of Brokenness.</u> Many were touched by the powerful testimony of both he and his precious wife, Dona after losing not one but four children to a congenital heart disease. Since that book was released in 2012, heartache hit them again. In October 2013, their grandson, Micah was in a car accident and was thrown through the windshield. Local paramedics after arriving on the scene immediately saw that he was dead but they were able to revive him while transporting him to the hospital. After 72 hours in a coma, despite around the clock care, and much prayer from family and friends across America, the Lord called Micah home.

How can one family endure such pain? It has been said, "Every rose has it thorn" and even Jesus, the Rose of Sharon was adorned with his share of thorns woven into a crown. Someone eloquently noted, "No cross without a crown" and Pastor Marvin and Dona Harris will have scores of crowns when they meet Christ in Heaven. What a reunion that will be for them with their Savior, children, grandson, family and friends who have already made it to Heaven! Micah was a remarkable young man with a bright future and he constantly had a smile for all and shined on the scene but served faithfully behind the scenes. He was an avid skateboarder and his heart was bigger than his body.

Just a month before the fatal crash he was with his grandfather at the Motor Vehicle Administration. While in line to get some information from the employee, he was curious what it meant to be an organ donor. He asked his grandfather what it implied and Pastor Marvin shared with him the specifics. Most teenagers are not thinking of others much less considering donating parts of their body to benefit another. After all, most are convinced that they will live forever never growing old. He asked his grandfather was he an organ donor? When he learned he wasn't, he asked "Why not?" When Pastor Marvin asked him did he want to become one without missing a beat he said "Yes! That's me!! Count me in!!!" When it was their time to approach the counter Micah said with a smile that he was going to be an organ donor.

The next few days and weeks, almost everyone he met he asked them point blank if they were an organ donor. If not, he politely asked why? For the last month of his life, it was his mission and this young man had a message. Perhaps Micah in his adolescence heard what President Lincoln heard as an adult and he knew that time was ticking and his days on Earth like sand in an hour glass was running out. They both knew what it meant to redeem the time and they invested it opposed to waste it. Death is hard but we find hope even in hurt. The Bible says, "To be absent from the body is to be present with the Lord."

The Lord called one of His favorite kids Home and what is still devastating to us here was and still a party up there. Micah had given his life to Christ just two summers previously at "Above and Beyond" summer camp. His leader for the week was a skateboarder at heart but a policeman by profession. It is so crucial to share our talents with others because a well-known preacher said decades ago, "God needs your personality." Your abilities and attitude will reach others that someone else may not be able to connect with. Some preach, others teach but we all must reach!

Since being ordained in 1998, I have officiated dozens of funerals and one of my favorite quotes to share is, "Some see death as a hopeless end but to the Christian it is an endless hope." What is the end for the lost is a transition to the saved soul. Pastor's wife, Dona Harris shared on facebook this testimony about her grandson, Micah just weeks after his passing on Earth and graduation to Glory. It touched all who read it and with her permission I am honored to share her words with you.

"Life is a precious gift. When our grandson Micah was on his deathbed, his decision to be a donor was honored. It didn't make it any easier telling him goodbye, but we were comforted somewhat in that his death would save several others. This evening I learned about four of the people his organs saved. Micah's tender, compassionate and brave heart went to a 47 year old mother of two who had been on the transplant list for three years. What a gift she has been given! Micah had a special way with kids. He would have been a wonderful father. He had so much love to give. Micah's liver was transplanted into a 51 year old electrician. He also likes mechanics and making things with his hands. Micah enjoyed those three things a lot! He was trying to decide if going into the military, a school for mechanics or perhaps a career as an electrician was his future. It is amazing that this man had all three of his inclinations and interests. Micah's left kidney and pancreas was gifted to a 41 year old woman. She was on dialysis for four months and had been on the transplant list for three months. She has been restored to her family and friends in good health. Micah's right kidney was transplanted into a 15 year old student from Washington, D.C. who had been on dialysis for five months and now his health has been restored. I wonder if he likes to skateboard!

Dreams have been restored for these people. They have been given a second chance to live a life they had hoped for. When our Pastor's wife, Lois Fitzpatrick, came to visit Micah in the hospital, she included in her prayer that the people that were receiving his organs would also receive his loving, generous spirit and that they would all come to salvation thru Jesus Christ. So, we are going to

ask that God answer that prayer. Then they will truly be
living the abundant life! We love and miss Micah every
day and are so proud of him."

The mother who was the recipient of Micah's heart has been invited to attend a future church service where Pastor Marvin and Dona worship. What a surreal and yes, sacred service that will be. It already brought health to her family and future but brings healing to everyone else left behind in Micah's death. What a reunion that will be! Micah indeed had a good heart in more ways than one and because he carried greatness he felt compelled by His Creator to share it. Thank God for the Micah's of the world who share greatness when most are content to bury it!

CHAPTER THIRTEEN

SPARING GREATNESS

D r. Johnny Pope in 1993 shared with me, "Frank, don't just keep the faith but share it." Two decades later those words have never left my mind. Greg Stier coined the phrase "Dare to Share" and I like it! When I was seven years old I gave my life to Christ. At age 10, in 1982 I had such a hunger for friends to come to faith in Christ that I brought 22 in one week to Vacation Bible School. The goal was not just getting them in church but pointing them to Christ. Later in high school the Lord impressed on me to host an evangelistic outreach in my hometown of Waldorf, MD. Several years after graduating the vision became a reality and with a nominal budget, audacious faith and help from a few friends, over one thousand people attended my first outreach at a local crusade. Go God!

The passages that gripped me while praying, preparing and promoting that outreach are found in Ezekiel 3:17-21, "Son of man, I have made thee a watchman unto the house of <u>Israel</u>: therefore hear the word at my mouth, and give them warning from me. When I say unto the wicked, Thou shalt surely die; and thou gives him not warning, nor speakest to warn the wicked from his wicked way, to save his life; the same wicked man shall die in his iniquity; but his <u>blood</u> will I require at thine hand. Yet if thou warn the wicked and he turn not from his wickedness, nor from his wicked way, he shall die in his iniquity; but thou hast delivered thy soul. Again, When a righteous man doth turn from his <u>righteousness</u>, and commit iniquity, and I lay a stumbling-block before him, he shall die: because thou hast not given him warning, he shall die in his <u>sin</u>, and his <u>righteousness</u> which he hath done shall not be remembered; but his <u>blood</u> will I require at thine hand. Nevertheless if thou warn the righteous man, that the righteous <u>sin</u> not, and he doth not <u>sin</u>, he shall surely live, because he is warned; also thou hast delivered thy soul." Some scholars may get hung up on translation but I still find the King James easier to memorize and grew up reading it since childhood. Regardless, the assignment is great but grace is greater than sin. People need the Lord!

Previously I shared about carrying greatness and last chapter sharing it but this is the thrill to some and tragedy for so many is to withhold it from others. We are instructed by God to share greatness, not to spare it. The greatest of all time is not Ali but the Almighty and when we share the Gospel (Good News) we actually are sharing not sparing Greatness and God in the process. Saved people desire to see people saved. Another translation may be found people want to help find people or one beggar telling another beggar where to find Bread. We had "lost and found" boxes in elementary schools for students to look for items missing but sadly too many churches have an atmosphere of entertainment more than evangelism. I am all for Christians having fun but it is no joke when souls die without grace. Defense wins championships but offense builds the Kingdom. When the United States Coast Guard learns of individuals stranded at sea they don't call them people but lost souls! It is interesting how the military got it right but many in ministry forgot it's all about souls.

God has allowed me to preach on all five of Praisefest Ministries cruises. We have been multiple times to Bahamas, returning for a second time to Jamaica in 2015 and Haiti in June 2016. We have witnessed over 39,000 souls repent of sin and trust Christ by faith. The founder, Dr. Matthew Dunaway asked me to be in a commercial to promote their "Water and the Word" relief effort. Several thousand Haitians die monthly because of E-coli and drinking water that is contaminated with bacteria

This time last year, Newton, Connecticut tragically lost 27 precious children when that senseless man entered a public school and murdered innocent lives. Picture that classroom times one thousand dying every single week! Praisefest Ministries has partnered with Global Effect and they have designed a state of the art water filter enabling people to bathe, wash dishes and clothes but most importantly drink worry free from the deadly toxins that have killed so many.

The video I was asked to film a segment alongside Josh McDowell, Dr. Johnny Hunt of First Baptist Church Woodstock, Tyler Perry's hit show "Meet the Browns" with Mr. Brown himself, David Mann and a few others! Initially, the plan was to fly me directly to Haiti to film on location. However, due to costs and by adding other voices to the project the green screen avenue made much more sense and saved several dollars!

My trip to Texas was around the corner. My dear friends, Pastor Larry and Shannon Baker at New Hope Church in Baltimore, MD where I have been blessed to preach several times said they had the green screen I needed to shoot the commercial. My four year old, Andrew and I drove the three hour round-trip in rush hour traffic to film. Shannon is a professional and we were out in no time. The film was forwarded to the proper media contacts for editing along with the other segments to make it complete. Instead of "3-2-1 action" we had "Houston, we have a problem!" Shannon said in all her years it had never happened before but the audio didn't record correctly and our efforts were in vain. She got straight A's for graciously willing to help out. It was discouraging but not her fault and we had to reschedule and do it all over again. It wasn't the end of the world but time was running short. My calendar was already on overload with a full schedule and even shorter for those dying (literally) in Haiti to get help.

Two days later, I had the pleasure to speak at King's Christian Academy in Callaway, MD for their Spiritual Emphasis and we had 34 students confess sin and profess Christ as Savior. Go God! On Monday, March 18, 2013 it was my privilege to board a plane and fly to Dallas, TX. That evening I was honored by "Olympian of the Century" Carl Lewis, nine time gold medalist and Dr. Sam Mings with the "Founder's Award" from Lay Witnesses for Christ for our recent involvement during the 2012 Olympics Outreach. The banquet was held at the gorgeous Dallas-Fort Worth Marriott in their grand ballroom at a black tie dinner in front of 1,200 at the annual Texas Christian High School Athlete of Year Awards.

The very next day, I had to catch a cab to ride twenty seven miles to Friendship West Baptist Church in Dallas. They have a massive 16,000 member church and graciously agreed to loan me their green screen and their staff to re-tape the Haiti project video. The hotel desk clerk when securing my cab shared on the phone that I am a preacher. I didn't tell her I was but she said that she could just tell when I initially walked in the lobby to check in. Praise the Lord! The man who picked me up was Muslim. I jumped in the car and as I sat in the back of the taxi I could see the meter on and dying to run. At first he was rude, impolite and even told me the price would be higher than what he agreed to on the phone. I was tempted to bail. In baseball terms, he had three strikes and I was almost out (of the car). However, those who display love least often need it most. God said "stay put" and we were on our way. The first fifteen miles, I let him do the talking. We talked about life, sports, business, politics and his family. I really believe when we LOVE folks first we can LEAD them from there.

At the sixteen mile marker I asked him about his faith. His reply made me curious. He said, "I am not a very good Muslim." I thanked him for his honesty. We talked some more and on my left side of the interstate was a Whataburger hamburger restaurant. If you have not been to Texas you may be unfamiliar with this particular food chain. I said, "Whataburger!!" He said, "Do you want me to pull over so you can get something to eat?" In all my years of trains, planes and automobiles I have never once asked a cab to pull over much less turn around and get me something to eat. For starters, when you live by faith you have to be conscious of the ever turning meter on the taxi dashboard. I have never found one to slow down or stop much less go backwards. Perhaps, I am *Frugal Frank* but he asked me again however we had already flown by the exit. I knew by turning around that was just adding more to the fare. This time, something was different. At this moment, concern for price was out the window. Not because I was starving en route to tape the video but I had a hunger to see this man consider Christ as Savior.

In my Spirit, the Lord told me to have him turn around and buy his lunch. So he turned around at another exit and came all the way back and we pull in to the restaurant. He said, "Do you want me to go to the drive thru or eat inside?" I asked him did he have ten extra minutes and he said, "Yes!" We walk in together and I told him to get whatever he wanted. He ordered a hamburger, large onion rings and Coke. I paid for our meal and now I am sitting across the table from my new friend (and taxi driver) and in between bites allowing him to ask questions. He peppered me with some spiritual questions and began to answer them in love with the help of the Holy Spirit. Talk about "fast food" God was serving up some soul food!

We got back in the cab and with just over ten miles to go I gently switched gears. While I was in the back seat staring at his rear view mirror I could read his eyes. It was as if the Lord gave me a window to his world. He looked anxious, tired and like he was running on empty. He was in his mid-fifties and he already told me he had a wife and two children who were more adults than kids. I asked him if he believed in Heaven and he said he did and I asked him to describe it to me. He said it was "paradise." I shared that I could relate. I asked him if he believed in Hell? His eyes got wide and said he did. I asked him to describe how he envisioned Hell? He said, "It will be a place of fire and torment." I told him I agreed completely, it reports that in the Holy Bible and he was surprised. From there I asked him how he could enter Heaven? He told me if he did enough for Allah than he might be accepted in. Politely, I asked if he died before he dropped me off at my destination what were his odds of going to Heaven? He looked down while driving nearly 70 mph and said almost embarrassingly "50/50."

God spoke to my heart and told me to ask him what did he think of those odds? He said, "Honestly, not very good." The next thing I said was without a doubt a dialogue between the Holy Spirit in me and His Presence that permeated the cabin of that taxi from then on. Knowing his eyes already looked weary and running on fumes I asked him if he ever lost sleep at night worrying about the future? He said, "Yes." I asked him if he ever stayed awake at night fearing of dying before the sun rose in the morning? He said, "Yes." I asked him if any of the stress in his life was tied directly to the fact that he was not certain that when he died that he would arrive peacefully at Paradise (Heaven). He said: "Yes! Yes! Yes!" In baseball, three strikes you are out! However, in bowling – three strikes and you are on a roll!! From there,

I shared that every other religious leader was still buried in their respective tomb. I told him in 1995 (age 23) that I paid nearly $3,000 of my own money to go to Jesus' tomb in the Holy Land knowing I would travel to see absolutely nothing. I told him the plaque on the tomb reads, "Why do ye seek the Living among the dead, He is not here but HE IS RISEN (Luke 24:5-6)!" I told him as Christians we don't serve a dead god but The Living Lord. He liked that!

Throwing the conversation into overdrive, I went from gradual to Grand Prix and when I saw the opportunity we went into over-drive (God and me). Faster than a Ferrari, I asked him if I could tell you that you could have 100% guarantee of Heaven would you be interested? His eyes while looking in the rear view mirror had me locked in like Tom Cruise in TOP GUN trying to shoot the enemy down. But this gentleman was no longer arrogant but available. He was no longer scheming for money but searching for The Master. He was still driving the car but God was leading the conversation. I shared in love but with Biblical boldness how Christ died on Calvary's cross not for His sins but our sins (including the driver). I shared how His sacrificial death, shedding of blood and Bodily resurrection paid the sin debt and by faith he could trust Jesus as his personal Lord and Savior. He would take our shame and clothe us in His Righteousness. We could graduate from religion to a relationship and according to The Bible in 1 John 5:13, "These things I have written unto you who believe on the Son of God may KNOW that you have everlasting life." I told him why "hope it" when you can know it!"

Just as the meter ticked that we had arrived at our destination. He was no longer looking in the rear view mirror but turned his head around to me in the back and said, "Will you pray for me?" I asked him if he were ready to confess his sins and trust Christ as His Savior and to be His Lord and way of life? He couldn't nod his head fast enough. This 55 year old man acted like a kid and by God's grace prayed with a child-like faith. In that taxi cab, he became a kid of the King when he trusted Christ. He even offered to knock off $20 from my fare. The irony is twenty seven miles before he was trying to raise it now he lowered the price. I recall when Jesus dined with Zacchaeus he said: "Lord, I will repay FOUR times for the wrongs he had committed." That is not only restitution but renewal and revival all in one! Hearing that Christians and clergy are often considered the worse in the area of tips I bought him lunch, paid the full fare and still tipped on top. Without question, when we LOVE others and LISTEN we can LEAD. Legalism is attempting to lead with no love. What the law couldn't do, grace gets done. When we go for the jugular first before getting to the heart of the matter (and stomach) we may miss out more than we connect.

Before flying home, I had the privilege to return for the second time and preach chapel at First Baptist Church of Dallas, Texas to their awesome students. We had three saved but over one hundred stream to the altar making various commitments to Christ and getting a burden for lost friends. I preached from Hebrews 12:1-3: "The Cost, The Cross and The Christ." I preached about The Crowd in the Cloud, Christ on a Cross and Christians in a Crisis. God gave me that outline years ago during a season of fasting. The day before, I was sharing about Christ, His Cross and Coming again to one individual but the very next day preaching chapel at the school to one of the largest churches in the country. They moved into their new $130 million facility on Easter Sunday of last year.

Immediately after the chapel at First Baptist Academy in downtown Dallas, I was whisked to the airport to catch my flight. This time I was not in a taxi but a car and it hit me like a ton of bricks. Looking in my rear view mirror I learned two things. What was a setback in Baltimore (driving three hours for a commercial that didn't have audio) was a set up from God in Dallas. Had the commercial worked in Maryland I wouldn't have been in a cab in Texas. Keep in mind when you encounter disappointment in the present it could be Divine Appointments for your future.

Plus, if we share our faith when no one is watching we will do it when a few others are watching. Regardless if on Trinity Broadcast Network (TBN) or in a taxi it is always an audience of One. That day on Facebook and social media I shared the news what God did and in one day received over 600 likes and comments on this event. It also reveals that it is sincere when we minister not just on stage but off camera in daily interactions with others on the road of life. The Great Commission literally means 'as you are going preach the

Gospel'. It is no accident that one of my all-time favorite television shows is Highway to Heaven. Every soul is saved one at a time and thank God for imperfections, Whataburger and U-Turns because God (like the water filter) truly makes the cloudy clear, the crooked straight and gives us double for our trouble. Thank you Jesus! Whataburger is one thing but WHAT-A-GOD is everything!

CHAPTER FOURTEEN

WEARING GREATNESS

We have talked about carrying, sharing and not sparing greatness but in this next to last chapter I will remind you that as born again Christians we are literally wearing greatness. The Bible says, "But we have this treasure in earthen vessels, so that the surpassing greatness of the power will be of God and not from ourselves (2 Corinthians 4:7)." Did you see that? The greatness of God is not because of us but deposited in us because of Him.

A friend of mine married one of the band members to Grammy Winners Jars of Clay and on several occasions I was blessed to spend some time with them, preach at one of their concerts, get on the tour bus with them, be a guest in their home and even recorded a brief clip of me preaching on a CD song selection by another praise band for their album in "Jars" recording studio in Franklin, TN that was eventually released on the radio! This verse above is the mission statement and motto of their ministry. The New International Version records that same verse, "But we have this treasure in "jars of clay" to show that this all-surpassing power is from God and not from us."

The Bible also reminds us repeatedly to put on the full armor of God. As a teen, one of my favorite hobbies was detailing cars. Nothing like washing and waxing an automobile and I found tremendous pride making an old car look new. One of my favorite touches to complete the wash was adding Armor All on the tires. Nothing like glossy paint and wet tires and that was icing to my cake. I often recall when holding the Armor All bottle was immediately reminded of that passage. Do you have the full armor of God on or in this case have all the armor on? In battle, the armor not only preserves but protects. It is a military fact if you don't wear the proper gear you can actually get demoted by your superiors and in worse case scenarios can be killed by the enemy.

When we receive Christ as our Savior we receive the power of the Holy Spirit indwelling inside us. The Bible talks about the Holy Spirit as not only part of the Trinity but is the Paraclete meaning our advocate and counselor. The Holy Spirit is both a Comforter and a Heavenly Helper. With Meadowlark Lemon, I am known as the parakeet but with the Holy Spirit we have the paraclete.

Prior to faith in Christ, this may be awkward for some but the Biblical fact is God didn't save us to make bad people good but for dead souls to live. Apart from the saving grace of God in one's life we are still dead men walking and have no hope of Heaven without salvation in Christ.

As Christians carrying greatness it is imperative that with the help of the Holy Spirit, we model Christ in both private and public. Dr. Johnny Hunt said, "The Christian doesn't have the luxury to be unkind." Pastor Rick Warren of Saddleback Church in California recently tweeted, "Anytime I'm being cross, I'm not bearing the cross. Impatience reveals a lack of humility." We cannot turn it on or off and we must reach out with the love of Jesus to all we meet. Time is short and we cannot afford to play games. Just like an appliance in the kitchen not plugged in we will not function properly or with power if we try to live in our own strength. We need to be tapped into the Holy Spirit at all times, asking for His strength and help. Apart from God we can do nothing. We are all walking billboards and when folks see you do they see a glimpse of God?

Life throws curve balls and pop quizzes come at a moment notice and if we are not trusting in God we will fail. It is important to be in an attitude of prayer and preparation at all times. Lord knows, I have had made more than my fair share of mistakes and was ill prepared for those pop quizzes. Thankfully, God grades on the cross and not the curve. His blood paid the payments for all my failures. In my line of work as a traveling minister and occasional Fox News contributor sitting idle is not my problem or idea of fun.

About four years ago, I was called on to speak at two funerals, tape two television shows, speak in two states and preach eleven times in less than a week. The movie "Planes, Trains & Automobiles" comes to mind and the one thing I'm never at a shortage of is PEOPLE. Not talking about the magazine but mankind. Just the weekend before, I was with my college buddy, Billy Griffin, walking in beautiful Fort Myers, Florida while in town preaching in the Sunshine State and two people stopped me on the street to tell me that we're friends online and they've been blessed by the ministry. Praise the Lord!

Three years ago while back at home my wife, Ruth and kids dined out on a Friday night at one of our favorite places in Southern Maryland. I won't name the place because everyone is entitled to a bad outing periodically. Typically, the service is first class and the food – First Rate! Thirty minutes after being seated the waitress finally came over and took our drink orders. Half an hour later we finally got our drinks. An hour into what should have been our dinner, Baby Andrew began to *cry*, Ruth began to *sigh* and I thought I was going to *die*. An hour and a half later (after being seated) most of our food came out but Ruth's was not ready. The Snickers commercial danced in my head: "Not going anywhere for awhile?" It has been said, "If Momma ain't happy…….." you get the point.

The kids were getting restless and I have the patience of Job but was tempted to get weary. What was supposed to be a perfect evening with the family, dining at one of our favorite places, was turning into anything but the ideal dinner date. Ruth took Andrew outside to calm him down because he was running on empty. My daughter, Hannah said, "Daddy, why don't you complain to the waitress when she comes back out." The fact is the service was super slow that night, the food was late and now my wife at this point didn't even feel like eating. I had two options: make a scene or take the high road. With the clock ticking, late in the game (dinner) and running on fumes emotionally our waitress came back and I thought what would Jesus do? She knew the evening was not the best and her eyes were hesitant to look at me as she brought the bill.

Some customers may have been tempted to demand not to pay for some of the food or get a free appetizer but tapping into God's grace I said to the young woman, "I realize tonight was not a usual evening for either one of us and it was just one of those rare evenings where everything that could go wrong did. However, it is not your fault. I could tell you guys were slammed tonight the moment we walked in and I admire you working hard and pray the rest of your evening is much better for you as you continue to serve your customers." From there, I proceeded to give her my debit card to pay for the bill and she walked away. My daughter said, "Dad, why didn't you let her have it? The truth is the service stinks tonight!"

Less than two minutes later the waitress comes back with our bill to sign and had this huge smile on her face. She said, "First of all, thanks for not yelling at me tonight. Second, I thought that was you when you came in but wasn't sure and when I saw your name on your card I knew it was you! She then screams, "You're Frank Shelton!! Now she has my and everyone else's attention in a six booth radius. She said, "You spoke at my church over fifteen years ago and signed my Bible and I wanted to thank you for the impact you have had on my life! I still read from that Bible on a daily basis!!" She walked away, my daughter's eyes were bigger than the plate on our table and my heart skipped not once but twice.

By God's grace, we encountered a pop quiz that evening and didn't even know it. Thanks to tapping into the Holy Spirit by faith and not acting in the flesh, we passed that test. Can you imagine how I would have felt if on that one instance (when the Spirit is willing but the flesh is weak) I had belittled that young lady? My testimony would have suffered and worse, may have hindered her walk with the Lord. In this journey with Jesus we don't have to be famous but faithful. When we wear greatness we will be a fragrance of the Father and have the aroma of the Almighty.

The next time you are hit with a pop quiz may you too dig deep and press into God to give Him Glory in both your victories and valleys. We just never know when someone is watching but rest assured, The One who matters most (God) is watching and may we be found faithful. In school we got grades but in life we need grace. Everyone has a bad day (even preachers) but may we be a blessing to others because we represent Jesus all the time not just part of the time. Our testimony is more important than our titles and the word testimony has "test" in it. Keep in mind a pop quiz is a mini-test to gauge how we are doing at the time. Pop quizzes can come any time. When I was in grade school the teacher issued them when I least expected it or was least prepared. However, our Teacher has not left us ill-prepared. We have a helper in the Holy Spirit. We need to stay prayed up in order to promote out the love of Jesus in our daily lives.

Earlier this summer, I was driving my wife's SUV and all of a sudden the center console that is affixed to the ceiling literally came apart and was dangling, and nearly obstructing my vision! With a hand on the wheel and the other trying to put it back in place on the ceiling while driving, I realized immediately it wasn't going to work. After pulling over and placing the car in park, I noticed that it was broken and my Duck Dynasty duct tape wasn't going to address the problem either.

My dear friend, Butch Hunt owns a local car dealership and is also a devout Christian. After calling him, I scheduled an appointment and prayed that the repair bill wouldn't be too steep. At the dealership, I caught up with the dealership owner's brother, Rick and he got in the car and indicated what I already knew - that it was broken and would have to order a new part. When I first heard the price for the part my heart dropped and I was thinking, all that money for a part that you cannot even see! He then reminded me that without the un-seen part doing its job it wouldn't allow the visible to do its job much less look good doing it!

The price of that part was a priceless lesson from the Holy Spirit for us all. Instantly, I knew a sermon illustration was in there somewhere. Those of us blessed to be in ministry are often "visible" and on some type of platform or stage. One thing that I have tried to remember and practice for years is not only to seek out the unlovely or unpopular but those whom serve unaware or under the radar.

Several years ago, I was invited to be a guest on Total Christian Television (TCT) in Marion, Illinois. They are the third largest Christian television network in the world. One thing I learned during my years in politics is to reach out to everyone. Regardless if they could vote or had a voice the fact is they all had value. I worked for a Congressman and my boss could work a crowd and connect with folks like very few others could. During my four years working for him, I also served a stint for just under a year as his full-time driver. I would drive to his home daily and then get in his car and drive him to Capitol Hill and wherever he went that day regardless if to Washington, Wal-Mart or The White House (literally).

Daily, I watched him carefully. I noticed he not only shook hands and made eye contact when speaking to the powerful and popular but with the poor, too. He would converse with leaders and laborers with ease and was intentional about it. It's impossible to be relational if you aren't willing to be intentional. The Congressman would be with the Provost of a University one moment and the janitor the next and yet made both feel important. That day on the set of "TCT" I walked in and to this day, try to picture not only Jesus in me but God going before. I picture Him connecting with each person and follow His footsteps. With that image of Christ in my head (and heart) I try to love on folks before, during and after ministering. Personally, I believe how we act off stage says more about us than when being on stage. Right before taping the show, one of the assistants from TCT "Rejoice" retrieved me from their Green Room and ushered me to their studio set. In my mind, I had a mental snapshot in part recalling my days with the Congressman but fully aware of Christ. At that moment, I began to say "hi" to each person en route to sitting -on their Oprah- like couch. As the producers were doing their last second checks before going live around the country on television, I said a silent prayer that God would use the interview for His glory.

As the camera crew adjusted their lenses and the producer counted down 3-2-1 and rolled into the intro with the theme song, the Holy Spirit showed up! God moved and it was an honor to watch Him work. When it was over, I intentionally said good bye to folks from the makeup artist to producer and knowing I needed to connect with the janitors before leaving the studio desiring to encourage them and thank them for their ministry, too. Heading towards the door, I spotted a woman who was running one of the massive cameras wearing a headset and I approached her. Fortunately, I recall saying "hi" coming in but wanted to say "bye" as I was leaving.

As she was taking off her headset, I was reaching out to thank her and I noticed tears streaming down her face. She was not even concerned about her mascara running down like Niagara Falls and she asked if I could step outside in the hallway to talk? I said, "Sure." We did and I was thinking perhaps the Holy Spirit said something through me that ministered to her or she wanted me to elaborate on a subject. After all, I knew we are carrying, wearing and I need to share greatness. Immediately, what she said next floored me and I will take it to my grave.

With tears running down her face she said, "Evangelist Shelton, I have been working on this set for a decade and it's been my honor to run this camera behind the scenes. However, I want to let you know that we have had some of the most respected and recognized names and ministers in America on this very set. As she sniffled and struggled to speak while she wiped away the tears looked at me in my eyes and with blurry vision said, "I want to thank you personally because you were the only one to ever thank me for my ministry." At that moment, we both were crying! The irony is she was "behind the scenes" so others could be ON THE SCENE and yet too many were busy ministering that they forgot to minister to fellow ministers on the way in or the way out.

This week, I was reminded of that car part in my wife's car. I complained that it was expensive (even though you couldn't see it) but God reminded me of three things. First, many who are first will be last. Secondly, to whom much is given, much is required. Thirdly, try to thank especially those behind the scenes because they are in the ministry, too and quite frankly, God uses them to hold much of us in place. If they didn't do their job privately some couldn't do their assignment publicly. It is a team effort. Today, be on the look out to compliment and encourage. It's free to be like Jesus but it's costly to be a jerk.

CHAPTER FIFTEEN

ADOPTION > ABORTION

My buddy, Dave is one of America's greatest apologists and has worked with well known Christian ministers and ministries. During dinner at the National Harbor this summer he shared a story with me about his recent experience and he gave me permission to share with you. Dave noticed a young woman leaving her first visit at the late term abortion clinic SW Women's Surgical Center off of Greenville and Royal. This is Dave's account:

> *When I saw her I gave her a friendly smile and asked her to roll down her window. "Are you having an abortion?" I asked. "Well, I am thinking about it," she said. I started to get a little nervous. Time was slipping. I didn't want her to drive off. What should I say? At 6"7, I am a big guy and can be intimidating so I decided to speak softly. "My name is Dave and I was wondering if I could talk to you for a minute." She told me her name. She wanted to hear me. I could hear gospel music from her car radio. I continued, "I just want to ask you to please choose life for your baby. I'll be glad to help you financially support your child. I have friends, who have been in similar situations and surprised pregnancies, but God provided a way for them and now they're raising their children." At that moment I could sense that I was surrounded by spiritual warfare, but I knew that "Greater is He who is in me, than he who is in the world."*
>
> *Out of nowhere, Jim handed her some materials about the Catholic pro-life women's center across the street with a cross. She hung the cross*

across her mirror and said, "Thank you." I continued to speak softly, "I don't know your story, and I don't want to make any assumptions, but I know that you were created by God who loves you and cares about you right now. You may have gone through some tough times, that I will never understand, and you may feel like abortion is the best option, but there is another way. God understands you and the baby is precious in the sight of God. At the moment of your mother's conception, all of your genetic information was determined when you were in your mother's womb. She chose life for you and I beg you to please choose life for this little baby in your womb." I paused and then asked her, "Do you believe in God?" "Yes." Can't you hear? I'm listening to Gospel music. I replied, "Ok, good. Let me read you the Bible. Here is what Psalms 139 says: "For you created my innermost being, you knit me together in my mother's womb. I praise you because I am fearfully and wonderfully made; your works are wonderful I know that full well. My frame was not hidden from you when I was made in the secret place, when I was woven together in the depths of the earth. Your eyes saw my unformed body; all the days ordained for me were written in your book before one of them came to be. How precious to me are your thoughts, God! How vast is the sum of them! Were I to count them, they would outnumber the grains of sand – when I awake, I am still with you. I continued, "These promises are for you and your baby. There is hope for you! Let me read to another passage that talks about John the Baptizer and Jesus being babies before they were born. Check this out…I quickly flipped to my Bible to Luke 1. "This was written by a medical doctor my friend. At that time Mary got ready and hurried to town in the hill country of Judea, where she entered Zechariah's home and greeted Elizabeth. When she heard Mary's greeting, the baby leaped in her womb, and Elizabeth was filled with the Holy Spirit. In a loud voice she exclaimed: "Blessed are you among women, and blessed is the child you will bear. But why am I so favored, that the mother of my Lord should come to me? As soon as the sound of your greeting reached my ears, the baby in my womb leaped for joy. Blessed is she who has believed that the Lord would fulfill *his promises to her!"*

I could still hear the Gospel music playing in the background. I asked her if I could pray with her. She said yes. I held her hand as the music played in her car. I started praying quietly but then fervently. I started praying that the Holy Spirit would come upon her and thanked her. Jesus shed His blood on the cross for her sins and I began begging Jesus that his young woman would fully trust Him and the baby would be saved. After the prayer, she thanked me. She said she appreciated it. From that moment, she had to rush off to class."

Presently, over 125,000 abortions transpire every single day. Read that again! That is horrific. More folks are concerned about the welfare of a whale stuck on shore than a baby that is murdered before birthed. Our priorities are selfish, shameful and downright sinful. The middle word of both "sin" and "pride" is "I." Until we graduate from self and be mindful of others we will only exist and never live. True living and love is self-less not selfish and a relationship should be based more on devotion to God than emotion to man or woman. It must be more about faith than feeling because the first is eternal but all else is temporal. If we started our unions on the bedrock of Christ more than in the bedroom of an apartment we would be much better off. That is not being self righteous but in love expounding the Truth.

The problem with sex before marriage is it's based on lust and not love. Lust is what we hope to get from someone but love is what we hope to give. Secondly, it's formed on convenience not commitment. Since untold millions engage in sex before marriage they are now faced with consequences and decisions that shouldn't have even entered into the equation. This may sound antiquated but there is no embarrassment from finding out one is pregnant after marriage. God honors those who honor Him.

Selfishness is a slippery slope and abortion should never be a form of contraception. Some groups talk about the "health of the mother" and her "rights" but what about the health and wealth of greatness of the unborn child? It's interesting that some political parties are against the death penalty but FOR abortion! That will never make sense to me. Just because it is out of our sight doesn't mean it is off God's mind. It was President Lincoln that freed the slaves and it is up to us to grant freedom to another. The greats didn't become great because they burned bridges or squashed life but because they gave of self even if it meant their death.

Just because one is wrong at the beginning doesn't mean you have to end the life growing inside you. Two wrongs will never make a right. In fact, it often keeps others LEFT out. Relationships (both personal and professional) cannot be built on selfishness. Similar to Lee Harvey Oswald's hospital room, we will always come in second or last. One cannot win when we constantly cut corners or compromise. Before his death, John Wilkes Booth, after murdering President Lincoln cried, "Useless, useless!" He is living proof that if we live for self we die useless and undone. Both Booth and Oswald killed presidents but we are just as guilty when we as parents murder our child(ren).

The good news is you can find healing for those whom have had an abortion and carry the enormous pain for terminating a baby and unfortunately know intimately the horrible guilt. Find peace in the fact that God loves you more today than yesterday. Ask God now for forgiveness and He will pardon you and cover your dark secrets like fresh, fallen snow. The key is to learn from that experience and decide now and forevermore not to participate in that death game ever again. We are better than that! You are better than that!

Until we learn to put God's ideals first and consider others more valuable than self we will be bankrupt in more ways than one. What happened to the people of character not long ago who had a chance to live by choosing abortion but they were willing to die to let the child live. Quite frankly, I wouldn't want to be committed to one who can't be committed to a child. We need some people of courage and integrity to live right and stop helping millions of aborted babies be left out.

Just because a baby cannot be visibly seen outside doesn't mean they are no less alive inside the womb. The baby kicks the walls of the womb to remind us all who is growing inside. Why personally choose a slow life of death because of guilt rather than select a life of grace now? A baby in the womb is a CHILD not a choice and if you truly want to play you must be willing to pay. Not for an abortion but adoption! Even better to grow up and become the parent we are called to be. In life, we may meet some illegitimate parents but find no illegitimate children.

Ironically, Dave had the integrity to offer to help finance and support a baby that wasn't his when some men who are responsible for the welfare of their children are missing in action. I'll never forget the time I was with a friend on Capitol Hill and he said: "I am so lucky!" I said: "Awesome! Tell me why?" He said: "Frank, I have four kids from three different women and don't pay a single dime of child support!" That may have been one of the saddest, sorriest statements I will ever hear. Anyone can be a father but it takes class and character to be a Daddy. Never let lack of money propel you to have an abortion. Better to have morals with little money than have tons of money and no morals. True prosperity is internal not external.

NFL football player Tim Tebow, Mariah Carey's husband, Nick Cannon, musical genius Beethoven and scores of others had mothers who found themselves in a bind and contemplated having an abortion. The world would not be the same without their contribution to society. On March 26, 2013 Billy Hallowell of The Blaze compiled a list of Hollywood celebrities who are pro-life. Actually, the list may surprise you but hopefully encourage us all to promote life instead of death. Hallowell wrote, "Jack Nicholson may have played the Joker, but his pro-life stance is no laughing matter." Live Action News noted: "As a pregnant teenager, Nicholson's mother was pressured to have an abortion, but she refused. This has shaped Nicholson's view on abortion, making him one of the few pro-life celebrities." Jack quoted in a 2003 report in National Review said, "My only emotion is gratitude, literally, for my life. I'm very contra my constituency in terms of abortion because I am positively against it. I don't have the right to any other view."

Justin Bieber is another and his mother Pattie published a powerful book last year sharing her personal testimony and faith in Christ. Donald Trump is also pro-life. His stance on it changed several years ago when his friend who is married learned his wife was expecting. At the time, he wasn't thrilled about the idea and seriously was encouraging his wife to have an abortion. Today, the child is the apple of his eye. His friend told Trump later that having the baby is the greatest thing ever to happen to him and them as a couple.

Super model Kathy Ireland is pro-life and has been a voice for the voiceless for several years. Italian songwriter and international singer Andrea Bocelli shared that his mother was misdiagnosed with appendicitis while pregnant. She was pressured by doctors and friends to abort. Fortunately she chose to keep her baby and we are all better for it. The rest is history.

Martin Sheen is also pro-life. He has shared publicly that despite being a liberal Democrat when on the issue of abortion, his views are night and day from many of his Hollywood colleagues. "Sheen has spoken out about his wife, who was conceived through rape," Live Action News writes. "Her mother considered aborting her and, after the birth, dumping her in the Ohio River, but in both instances, she chose to give her daughter life instead." Hollywood actor and political consultant, Ben Stein said, "For me the number one issue is right to life. I don't think the Democrats are very good on the right-to-life issue," he said on a PBS appearance. "People who think abortion as a reasonable method of birth control just are never going to get my vote." Country singer Kenny Chesney also is pro-life and countless other country singers.

Here are some other names you may recognize from Hollywood and around the globe who survived being aborted and fortunately lived because of adoption: Aristotle, Art Linkletter, Bo Diddley, Clayton King, Dave Thomas, D.M.C., Edgar Allan Poe, Eleanor Roosevelt, Eric Dickerson, George Washington Carver, Greg Louganis, James MacArthur, Jean Jacques Rousseau, Jesse Jackson, John Hancock, John Lennon, Josh Shipp, Lee Majors, Leo Tolstoy, Les Brown, Melissa Gilbert, Michael Reagan, Nancy Reagan, Moses, Nat King Cole, Nelson Mandela, President Gerald Ford, President Bill Clinton, Priscilla Presley, Ray Liotta, Senator Robert C. Byrd, Tony Nolan and God knows how many others. Indeed, adoption is greater than abortion. What the "stars" say is one thing but what the Son of God is everything.

President Ronald Reagan said eloquently, "It is ironic that all the people who are pro-choice had pro-life parents." Maybe we need to get on our knees and thank God for parents (albeit not perfect) who gave us a chance when they had a choice. You will never be a champion if you don't give others a chance. Be a builder of life not a blocker to death.

Personally, I would rather die saving life than watch another die so I could live. We have enough selfishness and we win when we promote selflessness. Without character or class, we would be no better than a cult leader who offered their followers Kool-Aid and they died while we could conveniently run out the back door. One may exist but you cannot live like that. Dr. Billy Graham said, "Until we are willing to die you are not ready to live." Every pregnant woman is carrying greatness regardless if they personally feel great. What if Mary would have aborted Jesus Christ? What if Elisabeth murdered John the Baptist? What if President Lincoln's mother aborted him? God help us!

An Asian student studying at Yale School of Architecture designed the Vietnam Wall upon which presently has 58,286 names of those lost in the war are engraved. Ponder this: if we designed another wall with the same marble dimensions but engrave the nearly 60 Million names of all the aborted babies since Roe v. Wade and create another memorial do you know how far the wall would go? The Vietnam Memorial goes towards the steps of the Lincoln Memorial but the wall honoring aborted babies would stretch from Washington, D.C. towards Camden Yards Baseball Stadium in Baltimore, MD some 50 miles away. That is not a homerun but we all strike out when we live less than for God's best in mind.

Is this the legacy we will have as Americans? Is this the caliber of our character we will be remembered by? A people who loved their toys but murdered their girls and boys? We can do better! We are on a decline personally and nationally because we have failed morally. We are going down because we failed to exalt the One above all. Historian Alexis de Tocqueville said, "America is great because America is good but if she ever stops being good she will cease to be great." God didn't design us to exist being mediocre but live magnificent and carry greatness. When we live right we will tap into a power to realize Greatness carries us.

Dave shared on the phone last night, "Frank, I honestly don't know what the young woman at the abortion clinic decided to do. I often wonder did she have the abortion or do the right thing and allow the child to live." Friends, today you must determine are you going to give birth to the dreams God impregnated in you or are you going to be content aborting His assignment for your life? God chose death for His Son on the Cross that you and I could LIVE!

Pastor Marvin shared with me about a powerful true story dealing with abortion. Ministry can be messy and he shared of a woman that carried immense guilt for years over her decision to abort her baby. She wondered like many others if she could ever find forgiveness from God? Her clergy said, "God is willing to forgive you for both murders." She said, "Two? I only killed one!" The pastor with tears in his eyes and love in his heart said, "Our sin killed God's Son on the cross. Because He is willing to forgive us of the first I am certain He is willing to forgive you of the second too." She confessed her sin, asked Christ for forgiveness and now a born again Christian. That is grace personified!

Keep in mind that adoption is greater than abortion and we must think of others more than ourselves. Yes, carrying greatness can be heavy but missing your Divine Destiny is deadly. You are not a lightweight but a heavyweight! Never let your insecurity or selfishness rob another of their destiny. Today is high time to finally stand up, move on and live anew knowing that you were created to honor God and serve others. The greats are gracious and you have two options: bury greatness or carry greatness. By grace, I chose the latter. You can too!

"I have fought a good fight, I have finished my course, I have kept my faith: Henceforth there is laid up for me a crown of righteousness, which the Lord, the righteous Judge, shall give me at that day; and not to me only, but unto all them also that love His appearing."
2 Timothy 4:7-8

How To Get To Heaven?

It's as easy as ABC's

Jesus said, "I am the way, the truth, and the life: no man comes to the Father but by Me." (John 14:6) Good works cannot save you. "For by grace are you saved through faith; and that not of yourselves; it is the gift of God; Not of works, lest any man should boast." (Ephesians 2:8-9)

Trust Jesus Christ today! Here's what you must do:

1. **ADMIT** you are a sinner.

"For all have sinned, and come short of the glory of God (Romans 3:23)."

"Wherefore, as by one man sin entered into the world, and death by sin ; and so death passed upon all men, for that all have sinned (Romans 5:12)."

"If we say that we have not sinned, we make Him a liar, and His word is not in us (1 John 1:10).

2. **BE** Willing to turn from sin (repent).

Jesus said, "I tell you, Nay; but, except ye repent, ye shall all likewise perish (Luke 13:5). "And the times of this ignorance God winked at; but now commands all men everywhere to repent (Acts 17:30)."

3. **CONFESS** that Jesus Christ died for you, was buried and rose from dead.

"For God so loved the world, that He gave His only begotten Son, that whosoever believeth in Him should not perish, but have everlasting life (John 3:16). "But God commendeth His love towards us, in that, while we were yet sinners, Christ died for us (Romans 5:8). "That if thou shalt confess with thy mouth the Lord Jesus, and shalt believe in thine heart that God raised him from the dead, thou shalt be saved (Romans 10:9)."

Through prayer, invite Jesus into your life to become your personal Savior.

"For with the heart man believeth unto righteousness; and with the mouth confession is made unto salvation (Romans 10:10)." For whosoever shall call upon the name of the Lord shall be saved (Romans 10:13)."

PRAYER:

"Dear God, I am a sinner and need forgiveness. I believe that Jesus Christ is the Son of God and the only way to Heaven. I believe He shed His precious blood on the cross and died for my sin. I am willing to turn from sin. I now invite Christ to come into my heart and life as my personal Savior. Thank you for saving me and taking me to Heaven when I die and use me for your glory now on Earth. In Jesus Name, Amen."

"But as many as received Him, to them gave He power to become the sons of God, even to them that believe on His name (John 1:12)."

"Therefore if any man be in Christ, he is a new creature; old things are passed away, behold, all things become new (2 Corinthians 5:17)."

WE REJOICE WITH YOU FOR THOSE WHO HAVE TRUSTED CHRIST AS SAVIOR BY FAITH. Email us Frank@FrankShelton.com to share your decision to follow Him in obedience and graduate as a disciple of Jesus. We are proud of you and praying for your new walk in Christ.

ABOUT THE AUTHOR

Frank Shelton, Jr. is fifth generation native of Washington, D.C. and resides in Southern Maryland with his wife, Ruth and two children: Hannah Grace and Andrew Lincoln. He was born on President's Day Weekend (February 20, 1972) and wanted to do three things with his life since early childhood: Politics, Preach or Protect the President. By his 35th birthday, he was blessed to pursue all three vocations. Frank worked nearly two decades on Capitol Hill (U.S. Senate, U.S. House, aide to Governor of Maryland) and volunteered at The White House Presidential Correspondence Office for two U.S. Presidents. He left completely "by faith" on July 27, 2007 to travel the globe as an evangelist. To date, Frank has been in 48 states and invited to preach in over a dozen countries. He was the International Evangelism Chairman of 2012 Olympics Outreach in London, England with "Olympian of the Century" Carl Lewis and Lay Witnesses For Christ and tapped in same capacity for 2016 Olympics in Rio de Janeiro, Brazil. Frank authored "Career vs. Calling" and co-authored "Blessedness of Brokenness" and a featured speaker for UPWARD Sports and Compassion International. He is also a Fox News contributor weighing in on current events and politics with a Biblical perspective. Trinity Broadcast Network (JCTV) picked him as the closing preacher for their 2012 telethon and preached live on their worldwide network in Santa Ana, CA and was a guest on their flagship program "Praise the Lord" airing in NYC in January 2014 to over 200 million homes. He speaks at "Iron Sharpen Iron" Men's Conference and twice booked to speak at Six Flags America for Faith Day.

President Jimmy Carter in May 2013, invited Frank to open up in prayer at his home church of Plains, GA and despite speaking 200 dates per year he is also a White House Press Correspondent for a Christian News organization and attends press briefings monthly in the West Wing. Frank serves on advisory board of www.CruiseWithaCause.org and they have witnessed over 39,000 souls saved and can be found preaching across America and around the globe on cruises, conferences, camp meetings, city wide revivals, colleges, chapel and churches. He has shared the stage with some of the most respected names in Christianity and shares HUMOR, celebrity impressions and the Gospel Truth. In a nutshell, he gave his heart to Christ at age seven and never got over Jesus. Frank's ancestor carried President Abraham Lincoln across the street on Good Friday, 1865 the night of the assassination. Frank's family friend was personal friends with the late Elvis Presley and was tapped honorary pallbearer at his funeral in 1977. Frank's favorite person outside of Christ in Scripture is Joseph of Arimathea because he reminds the readers and audiences across America, "We don't carry the 'King of a Nation' or 'King of Rock n Roll' but we carry "The King of ALL Kings!" It is one thing to carry greatness but entirely and eternally different when Greatness you.

Regardless, if sharing the Gospel on "HANNITY" to homeless, Hollywood or Capitol Hill's most prominent politicians he desires that everyone come to a personal relationship with Jesus, The Christ.

Visit www.FrankShelton.com
@FrankSheltonJr

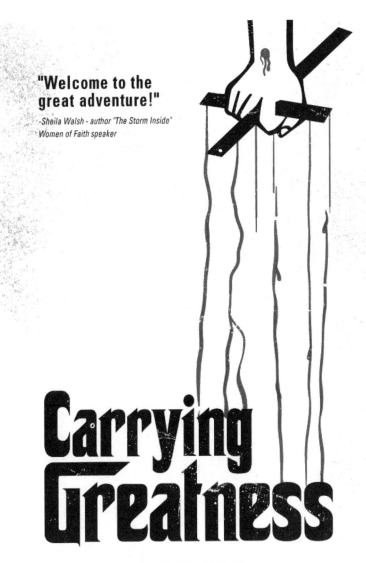

"Welcome to the great adventure!"

-Sheila Walsh - author 'The Storm Inside'
Women of Faith speaker

Carrying
Greatness

FRANK SHELTON, JR